# SQUAREDANCE FUNDAMENTALS

by John W. Jones
*Glendale, California*

Art by John W. Brinkmann
*Bell, California*

Cover by Chet Piotrowski
*Milwaukee, Wisconsin*

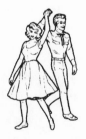

Published by
Jones Street USA, LLC
P.O. Box 610
Parma, ID 83660
USA

First Edition
First Printing 1971
Second Printing 2007

LIBRARY OF CONGRESS CATALOG CARD NUMBER 71-135474
ISBN: 1-4196-5981-2

MANUFACTURED IN THE UNITED STATES OF AMERICA

*Type set by the Alpine Press, Lake Arrowhead, California 92352*

*Printed by Times Mirror Press, Los Angeles, California 90023*

# TABLE OF CONTENTS

Unmarked maneuvers are Rudiments; those marked with an asterisk (*) are Other Elements. See page *xiii* of the Glossary for definitions of these terms, and Appendix A for a complete explanation of the definitions.

# FOREWORD TO THE BEGINNER

*Pictures and words*

This book explains, visually and verbally, 53 *rudiments* and 20 associated *other elements*. (See page *xiii* for definitions of those terms.) Together these 73 elementary procedures and maneuvers make up the bedrock base of modern squaredancing.

*73 building blocks*

All other figures, however complex, are made up of combinations of two or more of the 73 fundamentals. Therefore once you have thoroughly mastered these, you will be able to cope with any figure you may encounter.

*Bane of activity*

Of course there are many grabbag (catchall, or mishmash) calls nowadays. Each one of them is a "passel of pigs in a poke," as far as the dancer is concerned. Nevertheless, they are a current fad. So it will be necessary to find out what all is comprised by, say, "Squiggle Thru in a Scooby Doo."

*Must open up, find out*

But once you open up the grabbag and find out what it is stuffed with, you will discover there is nothing in it but an assortment of familiar faces. You then can deal with every pig in that particular poke.

*Anything know makeup of*

In fact, you should be able to do just about anything anywhere, as long as your memory for the contents of innumerable grabbag calls holds up. Meanwhile, you may be fortunate enough to dance to callers who are interested in providing you with stimulating, refreshing enjoyment, rather than a memory test.

*A delight to dance to*

There are some practitioners of descriptive calling (See Appendix C for details regarding this) here and there, and they are easy to recognize. They are the ones who are outstandingly popular—those to whom the dancers keep coming back month after month, year after year.

*Won't even hesitate*

If you should have the pleasure of dancing to such callers, you will seldom hesitate even for a moment in executing the straightforward maneuvers they call. For there are only 73 true fundamentals, and the simple "classics" or "standards" composed of combinations of two or three of them are not very numerous. Together, the fundamentals plus the few simple classic packages make up what are called *the basics*.

*Participation pastime*

Squaredancing is an inexpensive, extremely pleasurable diversion. Furthermore, it is far more gratifying than many other forms of recreation, because it is a participation pastime.

*As much action as like*

The action is practically continuous, and the dancer is right in the middle of it whenever he is on the floor—which can be as much or as little of the time as he likes.

*Your turn now*

Millions have enjoyed this fine group activity over the past hundred years and more; now it is your turn. Have fun!

# FOREWORD TO THE CALLER/TEACHER

*Logical development*

The procedures and maneuvers that constitute the bedrock fundamentals of squaredancing are presented here in a logical order of development, from the very most basic to those that are relatively advanced, but still fundamental.

*53 plus 20*

Of the 73 described, just 53 meet all the requirements of the definition of a *rudiment* found on page *xiii*. The other 20 are not rudiments, but are *other elements*, also defined on page *xiii*. They round out the full complement of elementary maneuvers upon which all of squaredancing is built. See Appendix A for full details regarding both terms.

*Categorized in appendix*

Each of the other elements is marked with an asterisk in the Table of Contents on pages *iii* and *iv*. They are listed in Appendix A and categorized in respect to the way in which they duplicate some rudiment and thus fail to be rudiments themselves.

*In functional groups*

Note that in the book itself the 73 elements are divided into 27 functional groups. This system of classification accounts for the fact that such apparently diverse elements as Square Thru and Grand Right and Left are found in the same category.

*May seem unlike, but aren't*

They may seem unlike each other, yet functionally they are identical. Both are pullby maneuvers. The only real difference between them is that one is performed in a small square pattern and the other around the full circle thought of as superimposed within the basic reference square.

*Okay with beginner*

The beginner comes into squaredancing unacquainted with its nomenclature and terminology. Therefore he has no preconceived notions regarding these matters. Hence seeing the two maneuvers mentioned above (or Right and Left Thru and Two Ladies Chain, or other pairs) appear in the same category arouses no antagonism in him.

*May not be okay with some*

However, many callers and long-time dancers have been accustomed for years to thinking of these things as being completely different. Some among them may not at first take kindly to what possibly appears to them to be a silly, thoughtless lumping of dissimilar maneuvers. Nevertheless, a little unvexed thought will show almost anyone that the functional grouping makes perfectly good sense.

*Up from scratch*

Furthermore, it is arranged in a logical order of development, being built up "right from scratch." Similar and associated maneuvers follow each other in ascending order of intricacy and difficulty of performance. For instance, the first functional group consists in procedures the beginner can carry out before he even learns how one walks in squaredancing.

*Usable in any way*

☞ **The contents of *Squaredance Fundamentals* can be used by the caller/teacher in any order whatever.** ☜

*Possible new plan*

The author believes it is feasible to develop a teaching plan radically different from all previous ones. That is, one utilizing the material largely in the order in which it is presented in this book.

*Would make easier*

Such a plan would exploit one of the book's greatest merits: its logical continuity. The continuous flow of one thing smoothly into another should enable the learner to almost effortlessly grasp the material and easily retain it.

*Will try it*

Whether it really is possible to teach the material in the order in which it appears here remains to be determined. The author

firmly intends to find out by actual trial, calling on the help of certain thoroughly competent, forward-looking teachers in the experiment.

*Helpful now; may be more so*

If such a teaching plan should prove workable, it would be as revolutionary a breakthru as the book itself. But in the meantime, *Squaredance Fundamentals* can be a tremendous aid to both the caller/teacher and the student regardless of how it is used.

*Hopes for the future*

May this most distinctively American of wholesome whole-family pastimes thrive for as many years in the future as it has in the past—and then some.

# PREFACE

*No change, just made clear*

This book does not alter a single entity in squaredancing. It merely presents the activity in a radically new light. In other words, the makeup of the pastime is not changed in the least, but is simply revealed in such a way that anyone can easily see its true nature.

*Experienced will see*

The beginner will not realize all this, of course, but it is fully expected that he will like what he finds here. The experienced dancer and caller, on the other hand, will immediately see that the presentation and explanation are indeed different from anything that has ever appeared before.

*Some will accept readily*

Some persons, because of their particular background of experience and their own personal characteristics, will immediately see the beauty of the approach's simplicity, be pleased and satisfied with that aspect, and accept the whole system on the strength of that one feature alone.

*Some willing to be shown*

Others who maintain an open mind will be somewhat uncertain but willing to be convinced if sufficient justification is brought forth to support the stand taken in the book.

*Some will be opposed*

Still others will receive the book with open hostility for any of a number of reasons. Primary among the reasons will be the mere fact that the approach is new and different. Some persons are opposed to new things simply because new things frighten them.

*Reason for appendices*

It is for the benefit of the second and third groups that four appendices are included in this book. In them inquiring persons are provided with answers to all their questions. Even the most dubious will find there solid, valid reasons, based on unassailable logic, for everything in the book and in the body of thought on which the book rests.

*Step by step*

In Appendix D a step-by-step description is given of the actual process by which the book was created, once the underlying philosophy and general approach had been established. Such matters often are of interest to persons inclined to be doubtful.

*Want to know process*

These persons are interested not only in the rationale undergirding the end result, but also in the manner in which the originator proceeded with his project. They want to be certain he did not start out with a good idea but go off on a tangent somewhere along the line while working out the final product. Skepticism of this kind is healthy.

*Problem and remedy*

Appendix C is an exposition of the true nature of one of the most pernicious practices in modern squaredancing—grabbag calling—and the simple, entirely feasible remedy for the difficulties it causes. The remedy is descriptive calling.

*Can help tremendously*

The author hopes that the key people in squaredancing—those in positions to actively influence its course of development—will carefully read all four appendices. For these dissertations can enable such persons to see that there are actually only a small number of true fundamentals.

*Will enable to appreciate*

The dissertations also will enable them to see thru the insidious lure of the grabbag call. Then they can hardly help seeing the beauties of descriptive calling and the tremendous potential it has for being a splendid stimulus to this fine pastime of squaredancing.

# HOW TO GET THE MOST FROM THE ILLUSTRATIONS

*Dancer views primary*

For nearly all maneuvers comprising a sequence of action, a series of dancer views is provided. In these the action is depicted as seen by the dancer himself—from above.

*Spectator views supplementary*

Certain maneuvers involve more intricacy of performance than do others. To provide the most comprehensible visual representation of these, a complete set of matching spectator views, as observed horizontally from some point on the dance floor, also is provided. Each spectator frame corresponds exactly to one frame of the dancer-view series.

*Compare corresponding frames*

To obtain the clearest understanding of the action, it is recommended that the reader examine first the series of dancer views, then the series of spectator views. Finally, he should compare the two corresponding frames (one in each series) at each point along the way, to see the correlation between them and grasp fully what is going on at each moment pictured.

*Unvarying in given series*

In a given series, the angle from which the spectator is viewing the action is unvarying thruout. But it should be noted that this angle does vary from maneuver to maneuver.

*Varies among series*

For instance, in a Right (Ordinary) Star Thru, all the spectator-view frames are observed from a position that is at right angles (90°) to the *right* of the gent as the pair begin the maneuver. But in the series for California Twirl, the point from which the spectator observes thruout is at right angles (90°) to the *left* of the gent as the pair begin the maneuver.

*Best viewpoint used*

And in the series for Box the Gnat the unvarying observation point for the spectator views accompanying the dancer views is very nearly *directly behind* the gent as the pair begin the maneuver. In each case the viewpoint selected was the one apt to convey to the reader the greatest amount of information concerning the action making up the maneuver and give him the clearest comprehension of it.

*The way the action flows*

Note that the order in which the successive frames of a series are arranged on the page is that in which the action flows. Almost all dancer views are delineated in respect to the gent, rather than the lady. To portray him on the page as he appears to himself and not oblige him to hold the book upside down, it is necessary to show him facing the top of the page.

*Advances bottom to top*

Consequently, showing him as he moves along in his customary natural line of motion straight ahead of him necessitates a frame sequence that advances from *bottom to top* of the page. At first blush this may appear rather strange, since the ordinary direction of progression on a page is from top to bottom.

*Unusual but better*

Nevertheless, a little reflection on the matter should show the reader that the unorthodox arrangement has great merit and is worth the minor "shifting of mental gears" requisite for his acceptance of the pictorial scheme.

*Sequence numbers help*

Very clear sequential frame numbers are provided to aid in overcoming the natural tendency to go from top down.

# ACKNOWLEDGMENTS

*Prime source*

First of all, I am deeply indebted to **ART STEINER**, almost ten years a fine caller for the famous Traildusters in Chatsworth, California—in its heyday surely one of the truly great squaredance clubs of all time. In providing practically all the basic information about the various maneuvers, he furnished me with the skeleton for the whole book.

*Indispensable consultant*

**GEORGE ELLIOTT** is known to thousands thru his "Elliott's Corner" writings for *Square Dancing* magazine. He supplied me with additional vital information and a proper understanding of all the material so that I could make the best use of it in presenting it to the reader. No less valuable were his mature, balanced comments and suggestions after I had gotten it onto paper.

*Additional help*

JOEL ORME of Canoga Park, California is another familiar "oldtimer" (in years of activity) among callers in the well-known San Fernando Valley. He was most cooperative in supplying odds and ends of information, expert opinions when requested, and anything else asked of him. In like manner, PAUL MAUPIN of Van Nuys endured a great number of question-and-answer sessions in an admirable spirit of helpfulness.

*Eminent counsel*

That "elder dean of squaredancing," **ED GILMORE** of Yucaipa, California, drew on his accumulated wealth of experience to make suggestions that led to the correction of certain deficiencies and enhanced the overall usefulness of the material.

*Essential adviser*

Another full-time professional caller known from coast to coast and popular all over the country provided yet a further check on the accuracy of the contents. **MARSHALL FLIPPO**, of Abilene, Texas, obligingly found time in the middle of a busy schedule to read the entire manuscript *twice*—once rapidly and once painstakingly—to make certain everything was as it should be.

*Wants to advance*

Still another full-time professional, LARRY WARD of El Segundo, California, is dancemaster of a number of highly successful closed clubs scattered along the entire length of the West Coast. He is much interested in raising the general level of styling, body mechanics, and other elements contributing to smoothness and beauty in squaredancing.

*Encouraging approval*

As an aid along those lines, he considered the material presented here sufficiently beneficial for his club novices to endorse it for use in his beginner's courses.

*All contributed*

These topflight professionals and others all contributed willingly and freely from their vast collective fund of squaredance knowledge to assure that the information contained herein was valid, widely applicable, and technically accurate.

*No passing the buck*

But the aid rendered by this impressive array of expertise in no way affects the assignment of the ultimate responsibility for the accuracy, etc, of all matters treated here.

*Responsibility author's*

That responsibility rests with me alone, and not with any of my sources or advisers. For in the final analysis (literal, as well as figurative), I am the one who is the compiler, coordinator, interpreter, arranger, arbiter, and explainer.

*Mr. & Mrs. Job posed*

JOHNNY and LYN MEYER, of the Traildusters, performed scores of maneuvers dozens of times each with Job-like patience while I took the hundreds of photographs (with a manual, single-shot camera!) from which the illustrations were drawn. Their equanimity in performing the maneuvers repeatedly, without music and oftentimes amid the throngs normal in a huge shopping center, was extraordinary, to say the very least. Without them there would have been no book, and I am profoundly grateful to them.

*Others before camera*

They were joined, for the two-couple and four-couple maneuvers, by GLEN and PEGGY ARTZ, MIKE and MICKEY PALAZZOLA, and JOHN and VELMA RIVES—all fine Traildusters.

*Deep appreciation for all*

My heartfelt thanks go to all these good people. Their genuine, unselfish interest in helping others to discover and share the rich enjoyment offered by our wonderful pastime was marvelous to behold. It was evidenced by the invaluable contributions they willingly made toward the birth of this first-of-a-kind aid for the square-dance novice and his teacher.

John W. Jones

*Glendale, California*
*20 November 1970*

# GLOSSARY

## General Dictionary Definitions

*element* — a component, feature, or principle of something; basic part; one of the relatively simple parts of any complex substance or process; one of a number of distinct units or parts composing a thing.

*rudiment* — a first principle, element, or fundamental, as of a subject to be learned; fundamental skill taught or learned (as in elementary school); a first step.

## Special Squaredance Definitions

*basic* — a fundamental or a fully accepted, very simple, and especially useful classic package made up of no more than three fundamentals.

*call* — an individual vocal expression (single word, group of words, or complete sentence) announced to the floor to direct one or more dancers to execute a certain maneuver or set of maneuvers bearing a single title.

*classic* — a single-titled maneuver, fundamental or package, that has endured in reasonably widespread popularity for five years (the period recommended by this book) or other period that may eventually be accepted by a preponderance of the policy-setting organizations such as callers' associations.

*dance* — (1a) all the activity of the caller and the dancers during the playing of a single piece of music; (1b) sometimes (in loose usage), the train of calls guiding the dancers; (2) a dancing event usually lasting several hours.

*descriptive call* — one that describes the action(s) expected of the dancer; that is, that tells him exactly what maneuver(s) he is expected to perform and gives him a fairly good idea of what is involved in his doing so.

*descriptive calling* — that employing only calls for basics.

*figure* — a set of movements; (sometimes) an action slightly more involved than a movement.

*fundamental* — a rudiment or other element.

*grabbag* — a package containing an inordinate number of fundamentals.

*grabbag call* — one having, usually, a single flamboyant title covering a package composed of an inordinate number of fundamentals; it commonly does not even tell what the constituents are, much less what is involved in carrying them out.

*grabbag calling* — that employing chiefly grabbag calls, oftentimes without helper calls; it very commonly masquerades under the misnomer of "high-level" calling.

*helper call* — an extra, additional call delivered after (usually) a grabbag call to make up for the lack of instruction in the grabbag call and help the dancer know what he is supposed to do.

*maneuver* — a movement or figure.

*movement* — simplest type of change in the positions of the dancers.

*other element* — a fundamental unit of activity differing from a rudiment only in being in some manner a duplication of some rudiment.

*package* — a figure bearing a single title but made up of more than one fundamental.

*procedure* — a particular way of doing something; method of doing things.

*rudiment* — a least-complicated process for accomplishing a most-elementary desired result; any simplest and distinctly unique action(s) making up a fundamental unit of activity; a rudiment always is straightforward and unembellished.

*train of calls* — a coordinated succession of instructions delivered in sequence during the course of a single piece of music.

# Notes

# SQUAREDANCE FUNDAMENTALS

## Group 1. STATIONARY PROCEDURES

## Attention

*Not a call*

The reader should note that the name of this procedure is never delivered as a call. That is, the caller never simply says to the dancers "Attention." Instead he says "Square 'em up," "Let's square up," or something similar.

*Takes action automatically*

In response to this sort of direct instruction, each dancer takes his place in the set and spontaneously brings himself to the stance of Attention, since the injunction to do so is implicit in the call.

*New designation*

The title Attention is one chosen by the author for convenience in referring to a stance that until now has had no formal name. The need for a noun title in talking about something is self-evident. It is hoped that this designation, along with several other mild innovations introduced for the first time in this book, will find acceptance among callers and dancers.

*Not military "brace"*

Attention in squaredancing does not mean the ramrod parade-ground carriage of the military, with chest thrust out exaggeratedly and chin pulled in grotesquely. Rather, it denotes a stance of poised, unstrained readiness in which the dancer concentrates on what the caller is saying and prepares himself to execute the maneuvers corresponding to the forthcoming calls. Good posture is an asset, though, just as it is in every other physical activity.

*Side by side*

Whenever a lady and a gent standing side by side and facing in the same direction are not otherwise occupied, they should join nearest hands, at or slightly above the gent's waist level, in the stance of Attention. The gent's forearm is horizontal or inclined upward very slightly.

*Gent usually on left*

Normally the gent is on the left; therefore he takes his partner's left hand with his right. There are a number of particular techniques that can be used for joining hands, but all are basically the same hold. However, they do differ rather markedly in the comfort they afford the lady, or gent, or both.

1

*Gent's palm vertical*

If both partners are to have the maximum amount of comfort possible, the "flat" surface of the gent's right palm should be absolutely vertical. That is, it should be facing directly to the gent's left. The hand is held in just about the same manner as it is in shaking hands.

*Lady's fingers drape over*

The lady places her left hand atop the gent's right hand. Hers is practically level, the palm horizontal and facing down. Her four fingers lie snugly against the inside surfaces of the gent's hand, her little finger in the smallest part of the vee **betwe**en his thumb and forefinger. Her **thumb** is held lightly against the upper **surfaces** of one or more of his fingers, on the **outs**ide of his hand.

*Gent's palm up no good*

If the gent holds his hand with the palm even slightly off vertical in the upward direction, his thumb gets in the way. Therefore his partner is forced to twist her wrist uncomfortably sharply to the left to fit her hand into his.

*Palm down unsatisfactory too*

The gent's palm can be off vertical in the *downward* direction almost any amount without making the hold uncomfortable for his partner. But even a slight amount in that direction makes it difficult for him to actively participate in the hold.

*Can barely grasp*

The reason is that his thumb is in such a position that he can only awkwardly grasp the lower parts of the lady's smallest fingers with it. Exerting such an ineffectual grip, his hand is little more than

an inoperative support for his partner's hand. Consequently, the hold usually does not have a feel at all satisfactory to him, since he is contributing so little to it.

*What to do with arms*

The lady can either let her right arm hang free at her side or use her right hand to hold her skirt out. The gent can let his left arm hang free at his side or can hold his left hand in the small of his back.

*Position of feet*

There is no particular position prescribed for the feet. Most ladies seem to prefer to keep them quite near each other. But the majority of gents appear to be more at ease with their feet separated a bit.

When a gent brings his boots right up next to each other, parallel and together, their midlines usually are separated by a distance of about four inches. So if he prefers to keep them six, eight, ten, or even twelve inches apart, the choice of a comfortable distance is his to make, and he will not look peculiar in his stance.

But when his feet get much more than about 14 inches from each other, he tends to take on a spraddle-legged appearance more appropriate to a stolid sentry on guard duty than to a lively, agile squaredancer.

Whether to keep the feet parallel or angle them out from each other is strictly a matter of personal choice. As in ordinary walking, most persons find at least a slight angle to be more comfortable than no angle.

*Lone dancer*

To assume the stance of Attention by himself, a solitary dancer (either gent or lady) simply stands erect, both arms hanging free at his sides, and remains alert.

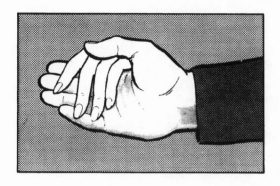

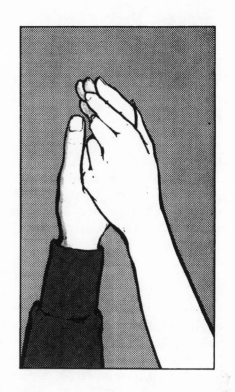

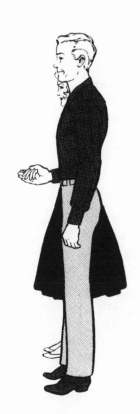

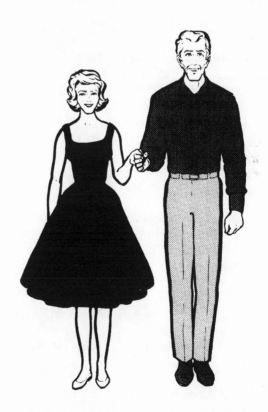

Figure 1.   Attention

3

# Honors

*Special squaredance use*

The term *honors* is unique to squaredancing. A plural noun, it has no singular. But the verb form *to honor* is used occasionally, as in "Honor your partner" (or other person).

*What honors are*

Honors are salutations, or acts of courtesy, in the form of bodily gestures. To render honors, each dancer addresses himself to a particular person of the opposite sex and presents himself in a formal demonstration of respect for that person.

*How and when rendered*

The customary ways of doing this are for a gent to bow and a lady to curtsy in acknowledgement. Honors are rendered by persons and to persons as directed by the caller—most commonly at the beginning or the end of a dance to one piece of music, but sometimes during it.

*Gent's arms, hands, legs, feet*

There are several things the gent can do with his hands, arms, feet, and legs in executing the bow. The most formal technique—the one this book recommends—is as follows.

*Other than his partner*

The gent holds his left hand in the middle of the small of his back, his left elbow out to the side. If he is bowing to a lady other than his partner, he holds his right forearm, horizontal, across and in contact with his midsection. The fingers curve around the left side of his body slightly. To aid in maintaining his balance, he thrusts one foot forward a bit, its heel about even with the toe of the other foot.

*Honoring partner*

His technique is essentially the same when he bows to his partner as they stand together. But first each of them takes one short backward step out to the side, away from the other, while retaining the hold between nearest hands.

As he takes his backward step out to the side with his left foot, the gent makes ¼ rightface turn (90°), pivoting on his right foot. His partner makes ¼ leftface turn as she takes one short backward step out on her side, pivoting on her left foot.

Thus they face each other, the lady's left hand still grasped by her partner's right. His right foot is forward of his left, and her left forward of her right, the proper amount for them to comfortably bow and curtsy, respectively.

*Customs concerning bow and curtsy*

The depth and duration of a gent's bow and a lady's curtsy vary with the area, the club, and the individual; but the action should be simple and unexaggerated.

Sometimes the gent's movement is not really a bow at all, but merely a sort of bobbing motion. Or it can even be no more than a distinct nod of the head. Even a shallow bow is greatly to be preferred, though.

Likewise, a lady occasionally will not curtsy at all, even though her doing so is very pleasing. If she does not, however, good manners require that she at least nod in recognition of the gent's polite gesture.

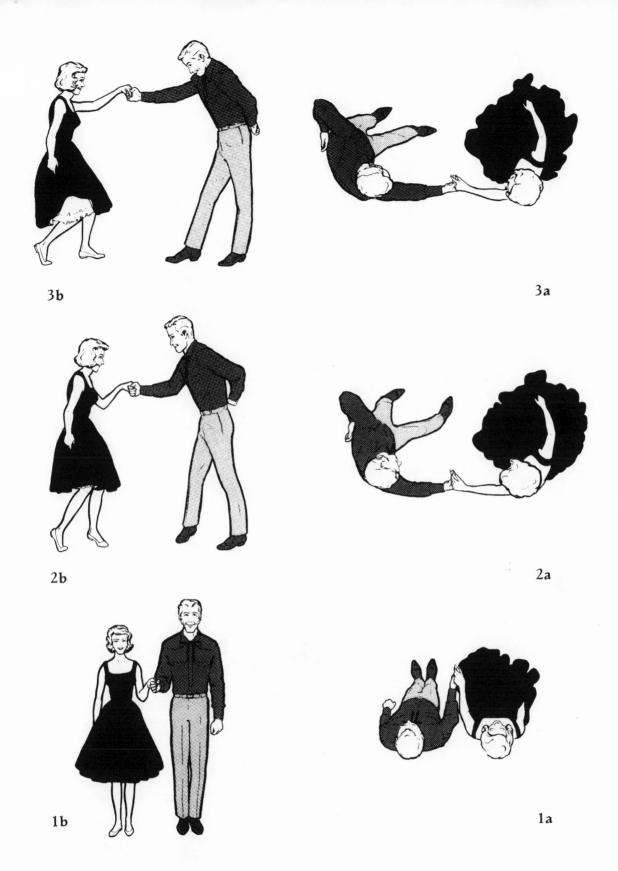

**3b**

**3a**

**2b**

**2a**

**1b**

**1a**

Figure 2. Partners Rendering Honors to Each Other

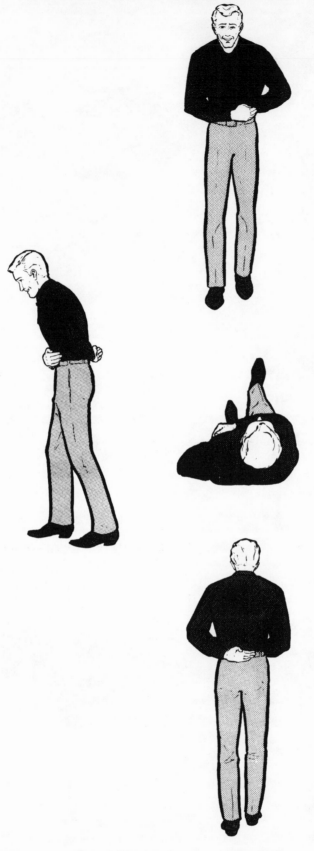

Figure 3.   Gent Rendering Honors to A Lady Who is Not His Partner

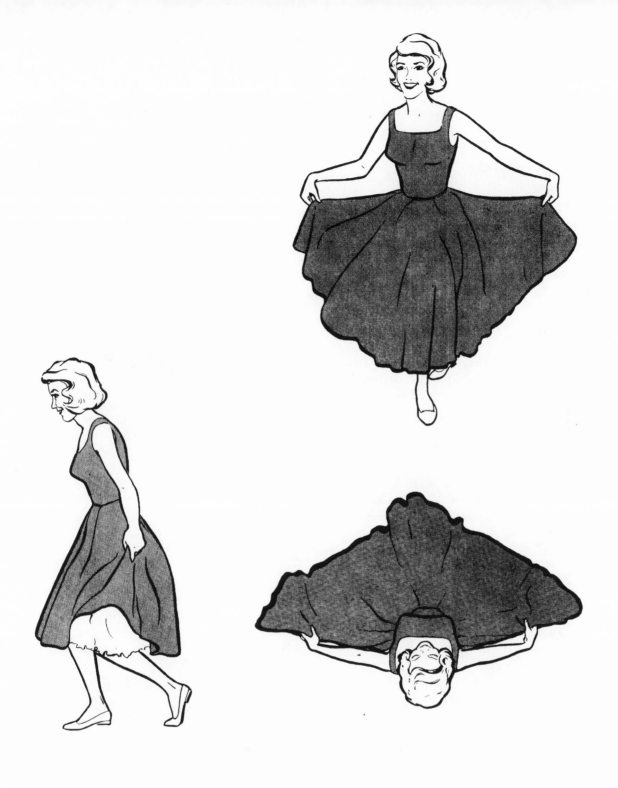

Figure 4.   Lady Rendering Honors to A Gent Who Is Not Her Partner

# Group 2. WALK

*Short shuffle step*

The step used by both gents and ladies at all times is a smooth, gliding, fairly short shuffle step to the beat of the music. Nearly all the weight is on the forepart of the foot.

*No up and down*

In modern squaredancing the dancer never at any time hops, jumps, springs, skips, bounces, or performs any other up-and-down motion whatever. Ideally, his feet at no time leave the floor. Whenever he moves he slides, slides, slides.

*Should strive for ideal*

In real life the dancer often falls short of this ideal technique of performance, and his feet do sometimes leave the floor. Nonetheless, he should not intentionally let them do so, but should diligently strive at all times to attain the ideal.

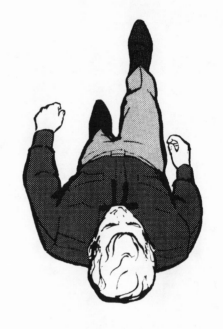

2

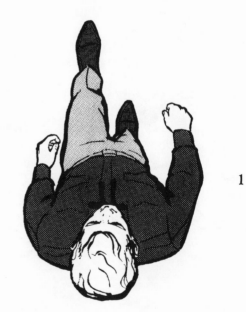

1

Figure 5. Walk

## Group 3. BALANCE

*Up or back as instructed*

This movement takes two counts (beats of the music) to execute. The dancer is instructed to perform Balance Up or Balance Back in accordance with the requirements of the dance.

*Usually one following other*

Most commonly he is directed to perform both, one immediately after the other. Usually the calls (delivered to the beat of the music) come one on the heels of the other and sound almost like one call—"Balance up and balance back."

*Sometimes separated or isolated*

Occasionally the caller delivers these instructions as two distinct calls separated by a beat or two of the music. In this case, of course, the dancer pauses between the two Balances. Sometimes he is told to balance up only, without balancing back, or vice versa. But such instances are very rare.

# Balance Up

*Step out, then "close"*

Stepping out with either foot (it makes no difference which one he leads off with), the dancer takes one shuffle step forward, then "closes" by bringing the other foot up beside the first, touching it or very close to it. He should perform these actions with an especially light and springy step. This sort of step can best be achieved by using the following technique.

*How to be buoyant*

As the dancer is bringing the second foot into position beside the first, to close, he smoothly lifts the heel of the first one a couple of inches, shifting all the weight to the forepart of the foot. He brings the closing foot into position with the heel already raised the same amount. Then he immediately redistributes some of the weight to both heels and allows them to sink to the floor rapidly and smoothly.

*Easy, though must be rapid*

This procedure must be carried out quite quickly. But the dancer should have little difficulty in doing so, because the process actually is much simpler to perform than the written description makes it sound.

The technique recommended imparts a great deal of verve to the Balance maneuver by giving a buoyant lilt to the dancer's motion in executing it.

9

# Balance Back

The technique employed in balancing back is precisely the same one used in balancing up, without any alteration except direction of motion.

*Step out, then "close"*

The dancer takes one shuffle step backward, leading off with either foot, then closes by bringing the other foot back beside the first. Even though he is moving backward, he still achieves the light, springy step in exactly the same way as when moving forward.

*How to be buoyant*

As the second foot is brought into position to close, the dancer smoothly lifts the heel of the first foot a couple of inches, then brings the closing foot into position with the heel already raised the same amount. The instant the second foot is in position, he allows both heels to sink to the floor rapidly and smoothly.

As in balancing up, this technique produces a buoyant rocking effect that is highly desirable.

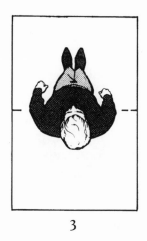

3

Figure 7.  Balance Back

1

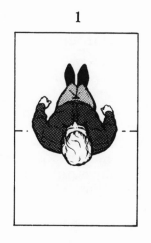

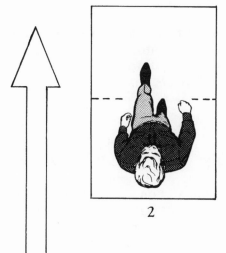

2

2

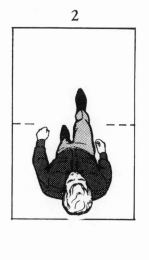

3

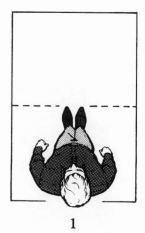

1

Figure 6.  Balance Up

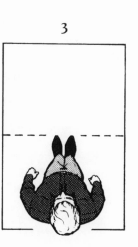

11

# Group 4. FORWARD (UP) AND BACK

*Use of parentheses*

The second word of the title of this maneuver appears in parentheses because although it is usually a part of the title, it is not always included. This way of indicating optional words in maneuver names is used thruout this book.

*Often performed by lines*

This movement can be executed by any number of dancers designated by the caller, individually or in groups. Most commonly it is performed by lines of dancers standing side by side and holding hands, facing in the same direction. Frequently it is carried out by two such lines, facing each other.

*Move in initially*

The dancers usually are positioned in such a way that they move in toward the center of the set initially. Whatever the arrangement, the maneuver is performed in the same manner.

*Up and back*

Using the standard gliding shuffle step, the dancer moves forward three steps and halts, then backs up three steps and halts. When he moves either forward or back-ward, it makes no difference which foot he starts off with. For ease in description here, we will arbitrarily say it is the left foot each time. A detailed description of the procedure follows.

*Forward three, then "close"*

The dancer moves forward on his left foot, his right, and then his left again. As he puts his weight on the left foot on the third beat of the music, he fixes the foot in that spot. On the fourth beat he "closes" by bringing the right foot up beside and even with the left one, fixing it there.

*Back three and "close"*

Then on the fifth, sixth, and seventh beats he backs up on his left, right, and left feet. On the seventh he fixes his left foot in position, and on the eighth he closes with his right. Thus eight counts (beats of the music) ordinarily are used in executing the Forward (Up) and Back.

*Can cut if necessary*

However, if the dancers are lagging behind the calls more than is desirable, they can catch up as much as four beats by cutting the movement down to as few as two counts each way: Step forward, close, back out a step, and close.

# Group 5. LINES

*"A line" in squaredancing always means a side-to-side row, never a column of one person behind another.*

## Ordinary Straight Line

*Standard use of term*

The plain word *line*, without modifiers, always means an Ordinary Straight Line. Such a line consists of two or more dancers facing in the same direction and arranged side by side, along an imaginary line thru their shoulders.

*Already in correct positions*

Invariably, the call to "Make a line of four [or six, or other number]" is directed to dancers who already are properly arrayed. To form the line, they simply join hands. As soon as it is formed, the line may move forward or backward, or it may remain stationary.

*Usual instructions about hands*

In practically all beginner's courses, the only instruction ever given concerning handholds is the time-honored one of "Gents' palms up [meaning way up], ladies' palms down." This is grossly inadequate, for different situations require different handholds—or rather, different varieties of the same basic hold.

*Hold for closely spaced line*

Members of a couple standing at Attention usually are rather close together. In this stance they constitute a closely spaced line of only two people. This short line is the most common instance of a closely spaced line. Hence the handhold best adapted for *any* closely spaced Straight Line or Circle (described later in this functional group) is called "the handhold of Attention." In it the forearms and hands meet so as to form quite an acute angle (approximately 30°).

*Hold for widely spaced line*

But when the dancers are widely spaced, their forearms and hands meet at a very open angle—something on the order of 120°. Consequently, maximum comfort is obtained by modifying the basic handhold. The gent rotates his wrist enough to tilt the "flat" surface of his palm slightly off vertical, upward.

*Thumb not in way*

Now the lady's hand can be placed across his, palm down and fingers across his fingers, in complete comfort. The reason is that if forearms and hands meet at a very open angle, the gent's thumb is not in the way when his palm is upward a bit.

*Lady's fingers drape across*

In addition, his thumb is better able to grasp her fingers, which can drape across his smoothly and comfortably, since they do not have to bend abruptly over a vertical stack of his fingers. Modifying the basic handhold as described results in a hold that feels better and is more satisfactory in general for a widely spaced Straight Line or Circle.

*Hold for circle of two or three*

Members of a very small, compact Circle of only two or three dancers find it best to use another variation of the basic handhold. For in this situation the forearms and hands meet along an angle so open as to be a straight line (180° angle), or nearly so.

*Fingers different*

Here the gent's palm (as shown most clearly by the back of his hand) is vertical, just as it is in the basic handhold of Attention. But his fingers do not curve gently out of alignment with his forearm, as they do in that hold. Instead they are bent enough to be completely at right angles (90°) to the line of his forearm.

*Gent's thumb angles across*

Also, his thumb is not straight out along that line, but is angled across the lady's fingers so as to grasp her index finger. Of necessity, her fingers are squeezed together a bit, but not enough to be uncomfortable.

*Only appears uncomfortable*

One could easily be deceived by the looks of this hold. It might appear that the lady's fingers are terribly cramped — so much that the hold would have to be uncomfortable for her. Rather surprisingly, though, it actually is not the least bit uncomfortable for either person.

*Lady's palm downward in all*

In all these three varieties of the one handhold, the lady's palm is in a horizontal plane, the "flat" surface facing directly downward. In two of them the gent's palm is vertical, and in one it is very slightly upward.

*One-third accurate at best*

Thus it can be seen that the stylized, standardized instruction "Gents' palms up [meaning way up], ladies' palms down" is at best a one-third-accurate description of the actual state of things.

*Standard instruction misleading*

It really is a disservice to the learner, since it is quite misleading. Which of these three varieties of the basic handhold is used is determined by the requirements peculiar to the moment.

*Tugging influences holds*

Here is one influence. In the efforts of the dancers to maintain the proper shape of the formation (linear or circular, as the case may be) and their spacing within it, they find it necessary to engage continually in a certain amount of hand tugging.

*Should be gentle*

Needless to say, it should be kept to a minimum and should always be gentle, never rough or violent. More of it is necessary in a Circle than in a Straight Line, because a Circle is much harder to keep in shape.

*What necessitates tugging*

The things that determine whether a dancer feels the need to tug, and how much, are the spacing near him at the moment and any deviations from the desired shape of the formation that exist near him.

*Different holds with hands*

Depending upon these factors, and perhaps others as well, he may employ a certain one of the three forms of the handhold. In fact, he very often uses one with his right hand and a different one with his left.

*Often change; can be intermediate*

A moment later circumstances may dictate that he change one or both. And of course if conditions require it, he may at any time (and often does) use a hold or holds intermediate between the three described here.

*Choice, timing not hard*

It may seem that the choice of handhold to use and determination of the proper moment to change to another is frightfully complicated.

In actuality, though, there is nothing to it, if the dancer has been supplied with the information provided here, and not just given the stereotyped instruction.

*Doesn't have to think*

Whatever holds the dancer may use, and however often he may alter them, he never has to consciously think about his actions. Without even having to practice, he does it all automatically, in the normal course of events.

*Comes naturally*

In other words, the foregoing account is merely a formal description of the actions involved in doing what comes naturally.

The dancer does it without even thinking, but only if he realizes the range of choice open to him. If he knows nothing but the inflexible "Gents' palms up [meaning way up], ladies' palms down," he initially will be ill-equipped to cope with the varying conditions he encounters.

*Will pick them up*

Even when he is left in the dark by being given nothing but the inadequate standard instruction, the dancer (usually after he no longer is a beginner) eventually picks these fine points up for himself.

*Produce of practice*

As he matures as a dancer, he comes into possession of these and many other niceties of squaredancing technique. They are body mechanics gained informally and unconsciously as fruitage of his continuing to *do*—to dance.

*Better if he is told*

But it is far easier for him to acquire and master these fine points, and it takes him much less time to do so, if he is *told* about them, instead of having to discover them for himself. Hence the detailed explanation here of handholds.

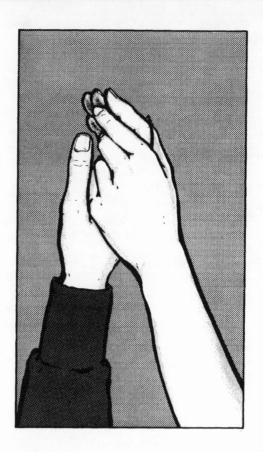

Figure 8.   Handhold for Closely Spaced, Compact Line or Contracted Circle

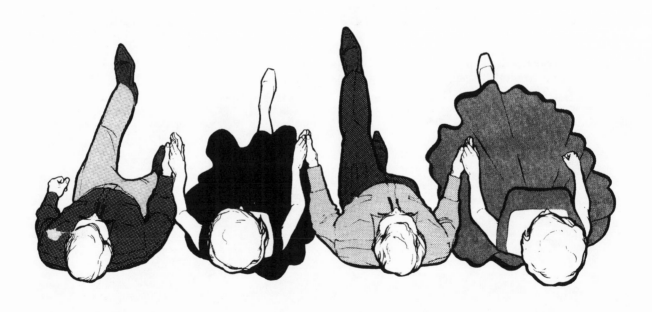

Figure 9.   Closely Spaced, Compact Line

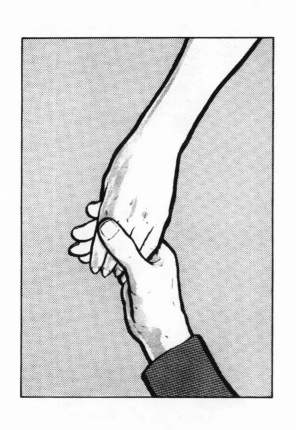

Figure 10. Handhold for Widely Spaced, Extended Line or Expanded Circle

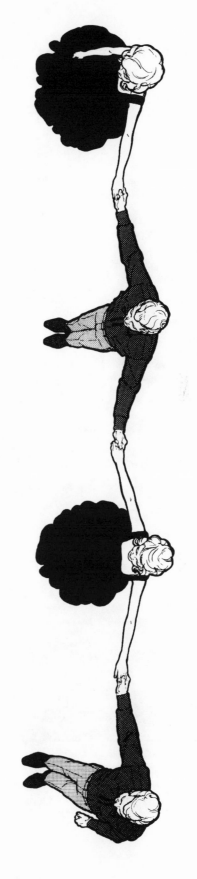

Figure 11. Widely Spaced, Extended Line

17

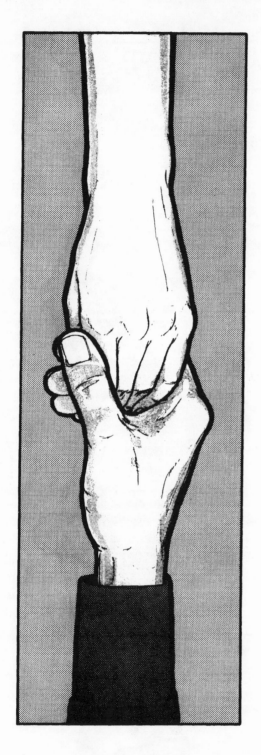

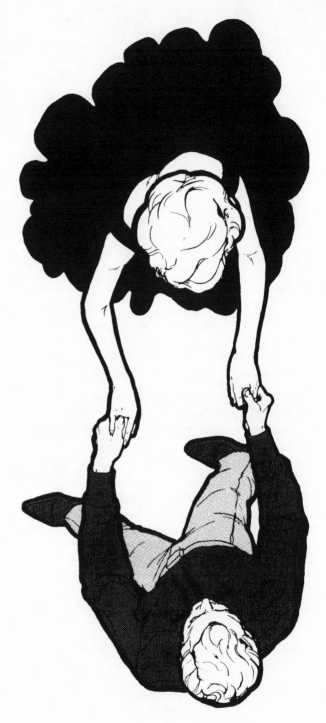

Figure 12.  Handhold for Very Small
Circle of Two or Three

Figure 13.  Very Small Circle of Two

# Ocean-Wave Line

*Opposite facing*

Thru the caller's selection and sequence of calls, three or more dancers are put into positions such that they only have to join hands to form a line in which each person faces in the opposite direction from the dancer on each side of him.

*Ahead one and pause*

When the caller tells them to "Rock up" (or "Rock forward"), they move one step ahead, each in the direction he faces, until all are shoulder to shoulder or slightly beyond. They pause in that attitude an additional count (beat of the music). Thus the rocking forward takes two counts.

*Back one and pause*

When the caller says to "Rock back," all take a step backward and pause an extra count. Each of the rocking movements is called an Ocean-Wave Balance. Rocking up corresponds to Balance Up in an Ordi-

nary Straight Line, and rocking back to Balance Back. In fact, those terms are sometimes used for the ocean-wave movements.

*Never two full arms apart*

When the line is rocked back, each dancer is very nearly at two-arms' distance from those whose hands he is holding. He is not quite that full distance from them, though, because he should always keep his arms bent an appreciable amount.

*No cushioning when straight*

For if he allows his arms to straighten out completely, there is little or no cushioning at the end of his travel away from the other persons. Therefore he is likely to impart quite a shock force to them when he reaches the farthest point and stops. This is rough, inconsiderate dancing that no one appreciates, and it should be carefully avoided.

There are two ways of holding hands in the line. Both will be described here.

## Conventional-Handclasp Mode

*At waist level*

This is essentially the same grip employed in shaking hands, at or slightly below the waist level of the gents. In order

that the palms can be forward, toward the other persons, the dancer has to hold his hands quite a way out to each side. Consequently, this method of joining hands produces a relatively long line.

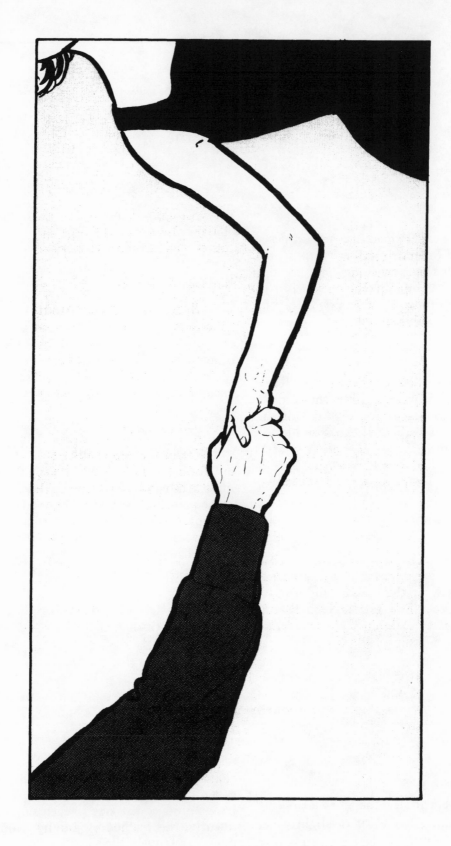

Figure 14. Conventional-Handclasp Mode for Alternate-Facing Lines

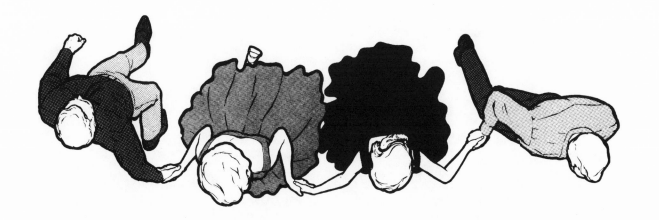

*a. Rocked Forward*

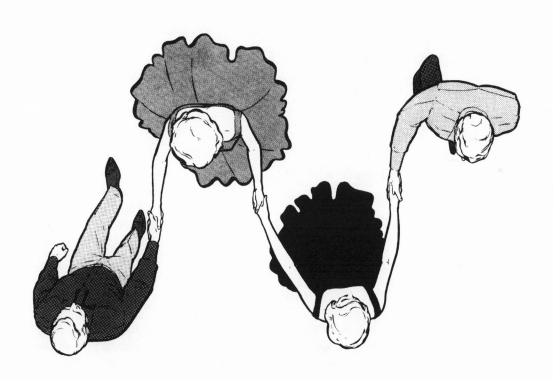

*b. Rocked Back*

Figure 15.   Ocean-Wave Line (Conventional-Handclasp Mode)

## Lifted-Arms Mode

*At shoulder level*

In this mode the joined hands are held at or slightly above the shoulder level of the gents. Fingers are upward and palms to the front, pressed together in a grip made somewhat interlocking because both thumbs are on the outside. When the line is rocked forward, forearms are vertical. When it is rocked back, they are about 45° from vertical.

*Relatively short line*

For the hands to be comfortably joined as described, the forearms cannot be displaced sideways very far. Therefore the dancer has to hold his arms closer to his body than he does when using the conventional handclasp. Consequently, this method of joining hands produces a relatively short line.

*Cannot step thru too far*

This mode offers one advantage over the other. With their arms lifted, the dancers are physically unable to "step thru" unduly when rocking forward. That is, they cannot step ahead inordinately far beyond the shoulder-to-shoulder alignment, as they can do in the handclasp mode.

*Everyone does it*

When they use the conventional handclasp, the dancers almost always step thru as far as possible. The practice is very nearly universal, and in itself is not necessarily objectionable, so long as it is done smoothly. But doing it violently is completely unacceptable, and the temptation to do so is always present.

*Pressure attracts*

The attraction lies in the increased pressure on the hands developed by the overtravel—it gives a heightened feeling of action. And, unfortunately, the more boisterous the stepping thru, the greater the pressure on the hands.

*Can be dangerous*

Any roughness is squaredancing is to be avoided. But the dancer should be doubly careful not to indulge in this particular type of roughness, for it carries with it a certain degree of danger.

If he succumbs to temptation, he runs the risk of straining his chest and shoulder muscles, or of causing the dancers around him to strain theirs. But even if no physical harm results, the lack of restraint is quite likely to detract from the other dancers' enjoyment.

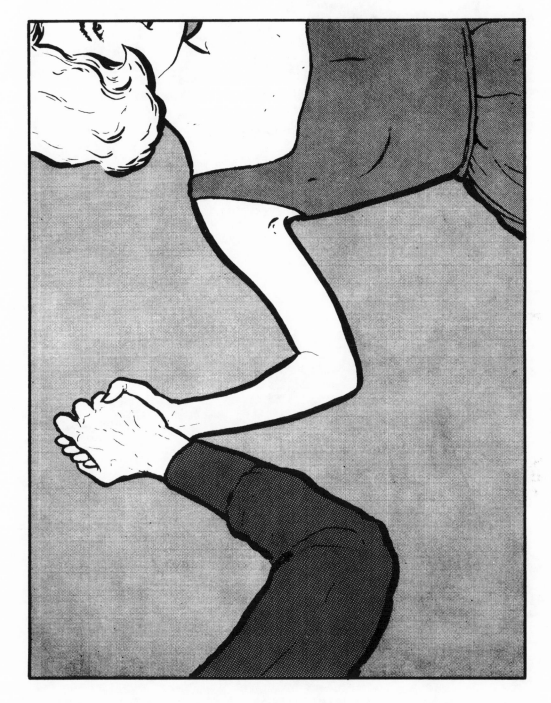

Figure 16.　Lifted-Arms Mode for Alternate-Facing Lines

23

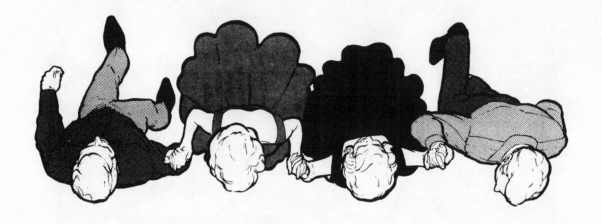

a. *Rocked Forward*

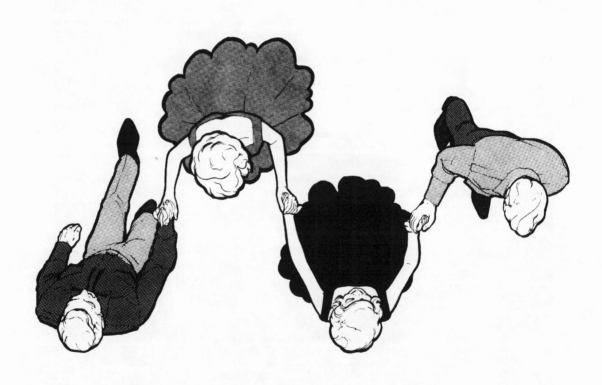

b. *Rocked Back*

Figure 17.   Ocean-Wave Line  (Lifted-Arms Mode)

# Alamo Style (Ring)

*Like Ocean Wave bent around*

An Alamo Style (Ring Formation) is in arrangement simply an Ocean-Wave Line bent around and joined at the ends to make up a circular formation. However, the Alamo Style is not established by forming an Ocean-Wave Line and then curling it into a circle.

Most often couples execute an Allemande Left (Left Hand Swing, explained further along in the book) in which each member, after he has turned halfway round (180°), grasps the hand of the dancer on his right.

*Opposite direction, grasping*

In an Alamo Style (Ring) a gent is facing in the opposite direction from the lady who was his partner in the maneuver immediately preceding the Alamo Style. He is grasping her right hand in his right. But interestingly enough, such is not the case in an Ocean-Wave Line.

*Same direction, one between*

In an Ocean-Wave Line his former partner is on his right, facing in the same direction as he, and is one person removed from him. That is, there is another lady between them in the line, facing both and holding one hand of each. This difference in arrangement in the Alamo Style and the Ocean-Wave Line results from the differing ways in which the two maneuvers are entered.

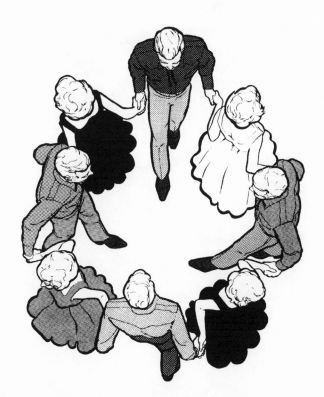

Figure 18.   Alamo Style (Conventional-Handclasp Mode), Rocked Forward

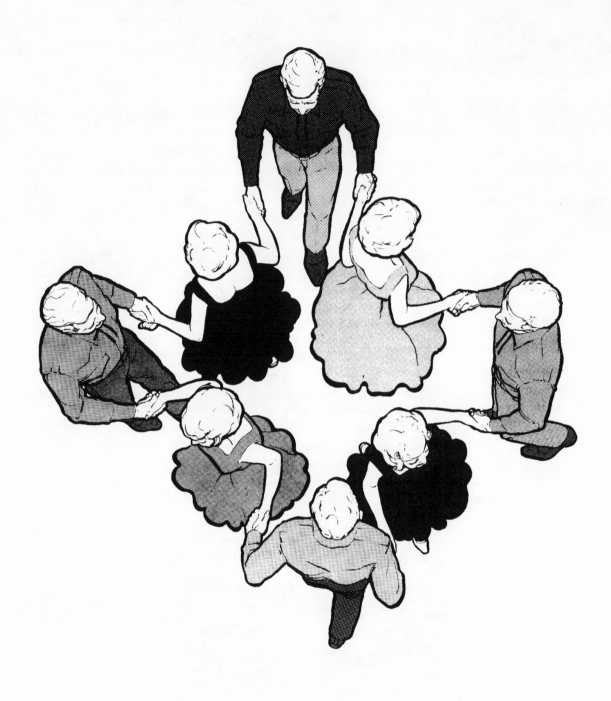

Figure 19. Alamo Style (Conventional-Handclasp Mode), Rocked Back

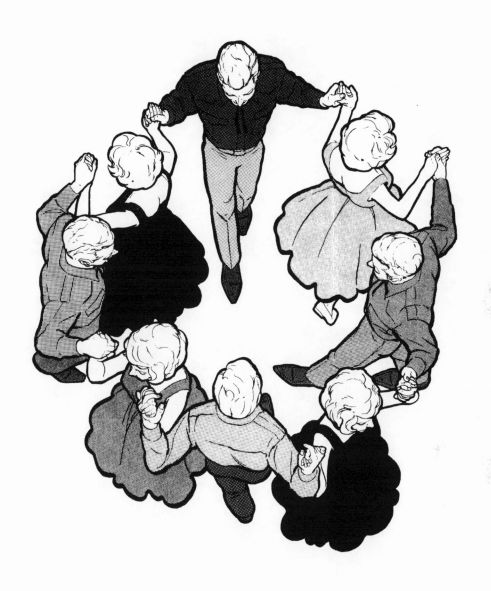

Figure 20. Alamo Style (Lifted-Arms Mode), Rocked Forward

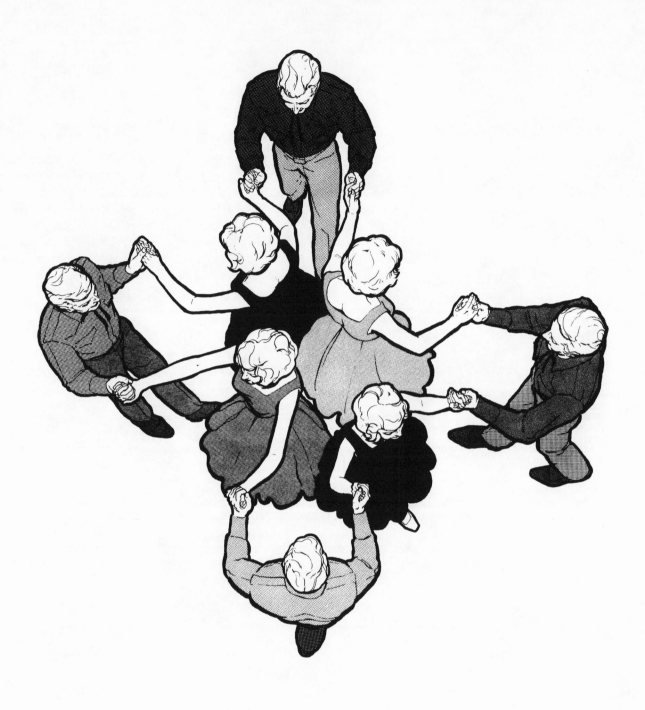

Figure 21.  Alamo Style (Lifted-Arms Mode), Rocked Back

# Circle

*Holds as appropriate*

The number of dancers specified or indicated in the call join hands to form a Circle (very often referred to as a "ring") in which all face inward. Handholds employed are any, as appropriate, of the three forms of the basic hold of Attention described in the first article in this functional group, on the Ordinary Straight Line. Each gent's partner is on his right, as usual.

*Normally move to left*

All move around the circular course to their left (clockwise, as viewed from above) unless otherwise instructed by the caller. When the Circle revolves in this direction, the gent's partner is behind him. When it revolves in the less usual "wrong-way" direction (counterclockwise), she is ahead of him.

*Don't move sideways*

The dancers do *not* move sideways (crabwise). Feet point in the direction of progress around the perimeter of the circular path.

*Body twisted to right*

When the dancer moves in the usual direction (to the left), his upper body is twisted to the right. That is, the left shoulder is thrust forward and to the right, and the right shoulder brought back and to the left. Only thus is it possible for the dancer to face (roughly) along the circular track and move forward around it while preserving his handholds with the dancers on both sides of him.

*Able to observe*

Maintaining this posture, the dancer is perfectly able to move his head around as necessary to observe the other persons in the Circle and coordinate his movements with theirs as the Circle revolves.

*Reversing direction*

If the caller issues instructions to reverse the Circle, the members simply slow smoothly and stop, then—without pausing—twist their upper bodies to the left, instead of the right, and proceed in the opposite direction in time with the music. Handholds remain essentially unchanged.

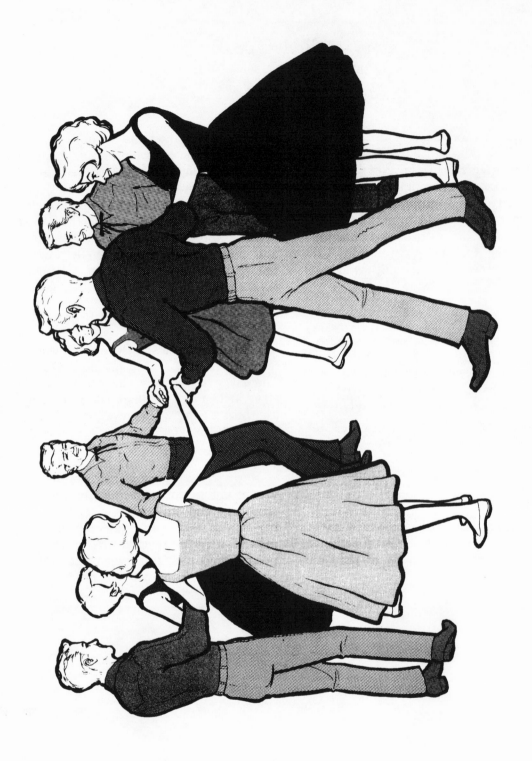

Figure 22.　Circle (Floor-Level View)

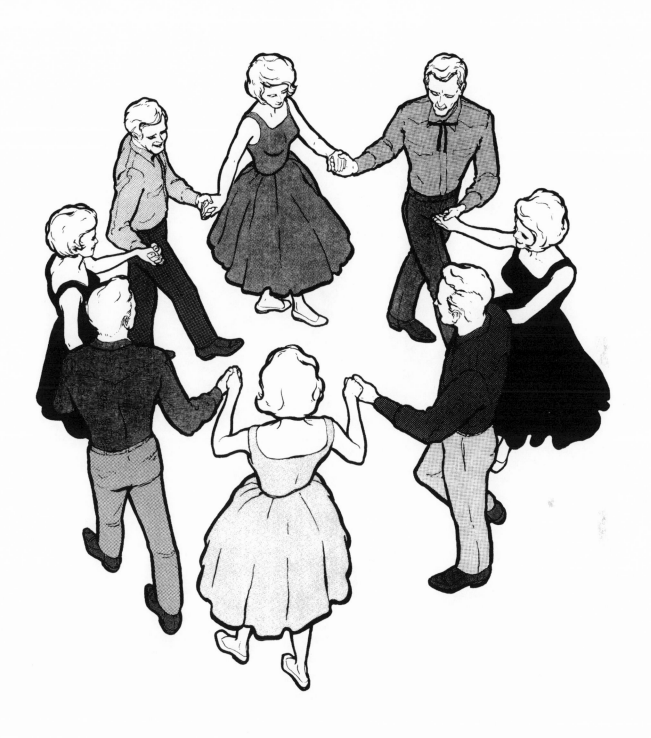

Figure 23.  Circle (Elevated View)

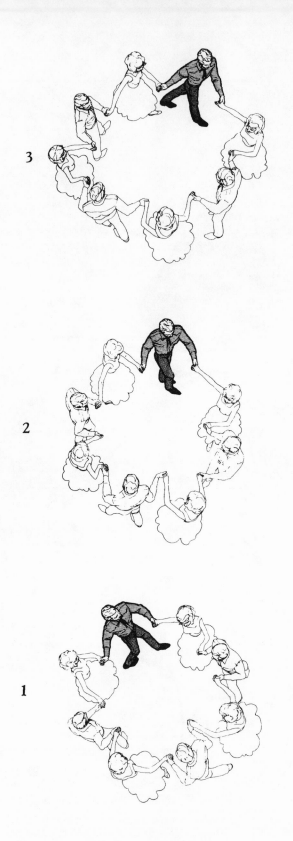

Figure 24. Progress Around A Circle

32

*Around inside or outside*

These maneuvers are carried out around either the inside ring, which is the inner portion of the circle thought of as superimposed within the reference square, or the outside ring (the outer portion of the circle), in accordance with the instructions from the caller. They are "lone" maneuvers in that a dancer does not perform them in joint, direct cooperative action with other persons.

# Promenade Alone

*Not a call*

The term Promenade Alone is a noun title devised by the author for convenience in referring to this movement. It is never used as a call directing the dancer to execute the maneuver. In fact, the calls always refer to the maneuver indirectly.

*Example of indirect*

For instance, "Number one gent promenade half" plainly tells that gent to promenade halfway round the ring. But it only implies that he is to do so alone, and not in company with his partner or anyone else.

*Normally counterclockwise*

Using the normal squaredance shuffle step, the dancer specified or indicated by the call walks around the inside or outside ring, as instructed, by himself. He moves counterclockwise (as viewed from above) unless otherwise instructed.

*Gent's arms and hands*

There is great diversity of custom in what a gent does with his arms and hands.

The easiest thing to do with them (and probably the most usual) is simply to let them hang free at the sides. But dancers in many clubs and many areas prefer a more formal carriage involving holding the hands behind the body in some manner. There are several ways in which the hands can be held.

*May be in small of back*

One way is to hold the backs of the hands against the small of the back. They can be crossed over each other. Or they can be separate, the fingers either together or spread out.

*Disadvantages of small of back*

The outstanding disadvantage of this technique is that the elbows tend to stick out quite a way and look ugly. But even worse, really, is the fact that they are a hindrance to the gent—and a danger to others—in close quarters. To prevent this difficulty, the gent must pull his elbows back, and doing so is not particularly comfortable.

*May be on hip pockets*

For this reason, quite a few gents prefer to hold the backs of their hands against their hip pockets. When the hands are that low, the elbows do not stick out as much as when the hands are in the small of the back.

*More comfortable*

Therefore this posture is a more comfortable one, since the gent has to pull his elbows back less, or perhaps not at all. However, there is a decided tendency to thrust the head and shoulders forward, creating a stoopshouldered effect.

*Note what others are doing*

Any arrangement of the hands and arms is acceptable as long as it does not have an unnatural, affected look. However, since squaredancing is a group activity, the gent would do well to note what technique most of the other gents around him are employing, then consider using the same one—or at least one that is not conspicuously incongruous.

*Lady works skirt*

Regardless of what a gent may choose to do with his hands and arms, it is a good idea for a lady to use her hands to whip her skirt back and forth, thus creating a vivacious, saucy appearance. She should, of course, do this in moderation and in a ladylike manner, not boisterously.

*Several may promenade alone*

Even though this maneuver is a lone promenade and is called Promenade Alone, it sometimes is executed by more than one dancer at a time. For instance, a gent may be instructed to proceed clockwise, and his partner counterclockwise.

*Each independent*

In such an event, however, each moves as an independent agent along his own course. Each dancer executing a Cross Trail (described later in the book) actually is in a special kind of Promenade Alone, even though his partner moves along beside him. The same might be said of Pass Thru (also described later) if the partners are not holding hands as they begin.

# Promenade In Single File

*Like Promenade Alone*

This movement also has the name Promenade, (Go) Indian Style. In technique it is identical with Promenade Alone. It differs from it only in that two or more dancers promenade in that fashion *as a group.*

*Counterclockwise normally*

They form a column, one dancer behind another and all headed in the same direction around the inside or the outside ring. They move counterclockwise unless told to do otherwise.

*Gent usually behind partner*

Moving thus, each gent is *behind* his partner if both members of the couple are engaged in the maneuver. In the somewhat less common "wrongway" clockwise promenading he is ahead of her if both are active.

*Sometimes only one active*

However, oftentimes only one member of each couple is active, as for example in responding to the call "Four ladies (or gents) promenade [in single file]."

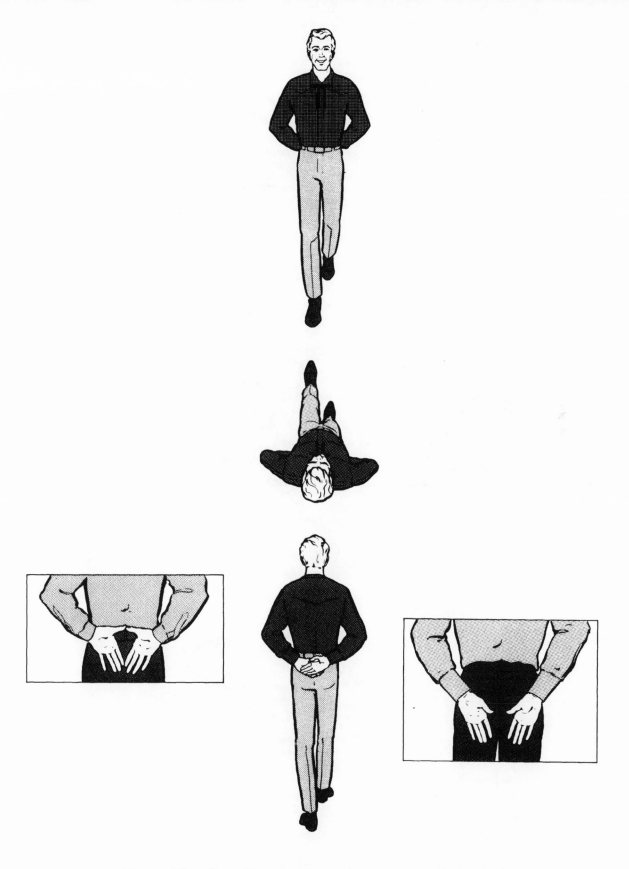

Figure 25.   Gent Promenading Alone or in Single File

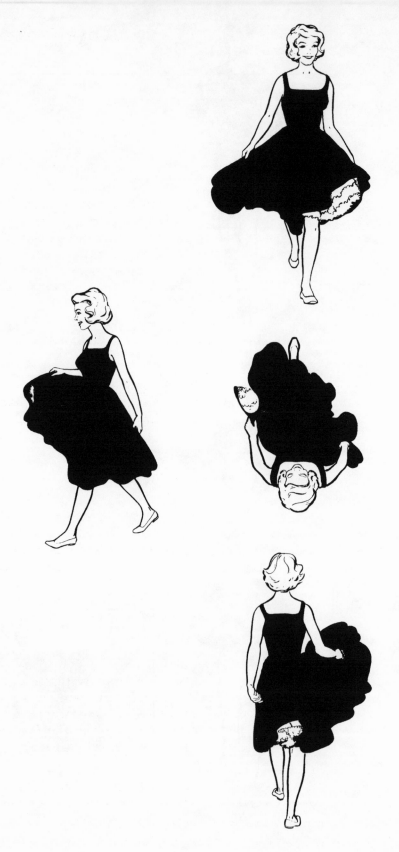

Figure 26.  Lady Promenading Alone or in Single File

# Turnback

*Prevalent instructions*

Because of a lack of standardization, there still is a certain amount of confusion concerning terms indicating a reversal of direction along exactly the same path by individual dancers. The two most usual instructions for such a movement are "You turn back" and "Make a U turn back."

*Fine as calls*

Both instructions are short, distinct, and rhythmical, in addition to being plain and clear in telling the dancer what he is expected to do. Therefore either is excellent as a *call*—an instruction.

*No titles till now*

But till now the most prevalent *names* for this movement have been rather inept. Quite commonly one or the other of the two *instructions* has been pressed into service as a name. Oftentimes a combination has been used: U (or You) Turn Back.

*Meaning clear but term awkward*

In any of the three forms, the meaning is clear enough, but as *titles* designating *the movement itself*, all three terms are awkward.

*New name proposed*

Therefore this book proposes they be replaced in that application by the designation heading this article: Turnback. Thus when the caller says to the dancer "Make a U turn back" or (in the sense presently under consideration) "You turn back," the maneuver the dancer executes in response will be a Turnback.

*Can mean two things*

But the reader should understand that the instruction "[You] turn back" currently can mean either of two things. Sometimes it means for the dancer to execute a Turnback as an independent agent, in the manner just referred to. An example is "Gents [, you] turn back."

*Other meaning*

Probably just as often, though, it means that the dancer is to execute a Forearm or Hand Swing ("turn"; described further along in the book) with another dancer during the performance of a more complex figure.

*One specific application*

For instance, oftentimes during the execution of a Grand Right and Left (described later), the call will be given "When you meet your partner, you turn back (or turn right back)." This tells them to swing halfway round so that each reverses direction and goes back the opposite way.

*"Double turnback" confusing*

The call "When you meet your partner, do a double turn back" means exactly the same thing. It does *not* mean that each dancer executes a Forearm Swing with his partner, then a second one with someone else.

Nor does it mean that partners swing full around, instead of half around.

This particular wording of the call is rather poor, since it is misleading. It merely is an inept attempt to emphasize the fact that each of the two partners performs, in effect, a Turnback in swinging halfway round in the Forearm Swing.

*"Turn back one [or other number]"*

Sometimes the call is "When you meet your partner, turn back one [or two, or other number]." In this event each dancer, after swinging round, goes back the opposite way to the first person he meets, the second one, or whichever one is specified in the call. Before he reaches that person, he will receive instructions as to what to do with him.

*"Turn alone"*

The call "Turn alone" usually is delivered to couples. However, it is directed *not* to the couples *as units,* but to the individual members of the couples. Each performs a Turnback independently.

*"Turn back" to couples*

Some callers do occasionally direct the call "Turn back" to couples when they want them to execute a Wheelaround (described later), although this is generally considered bad practice.

*"Backtrack" to individuals*

Also, some callers occasionally address the call "Backtrack" to individual dancers when they want them to perform a Turnback. But it is not good practice, because the Backtrack maneuver (described at its own entry further on in the book) is one that can legitimately be executed only by a promenading couple.

*"Reverse back"*

The call "Reverse back" is practically an all-purpose one applied indiscriminately to individuals, couples, and larger groups to cause them to reverse their direction of travel.

*Lone Turnback from straight path*

When an individual dancer is promenading in a straight line, alone or in single file, and is directed to execute a Turnback, there is no prescribed direction in which he is supposed to pivot. He may turn to either his right or his left in reversing his direction along exactly the same path.

*From parallel straight paths*

But a gent may be moving parallel with a lady, though, as in "Cross trail, you turn back." In such a case both common courtesy and the practical consideration of keeping the lady in view dictate that he turn *toward* her, rather than away from her.

*From circular path*

Similarly, the dancer may be in a circular or rotary formation and be told to perform a Turnback. If so, this book recommends he turn toward the *inside* of the set, rather than the outside.

The reason is that by doing so he can keep the other dancers within his field of vision while he is turning, whereas he cannot if he turns toward the outside of the set.

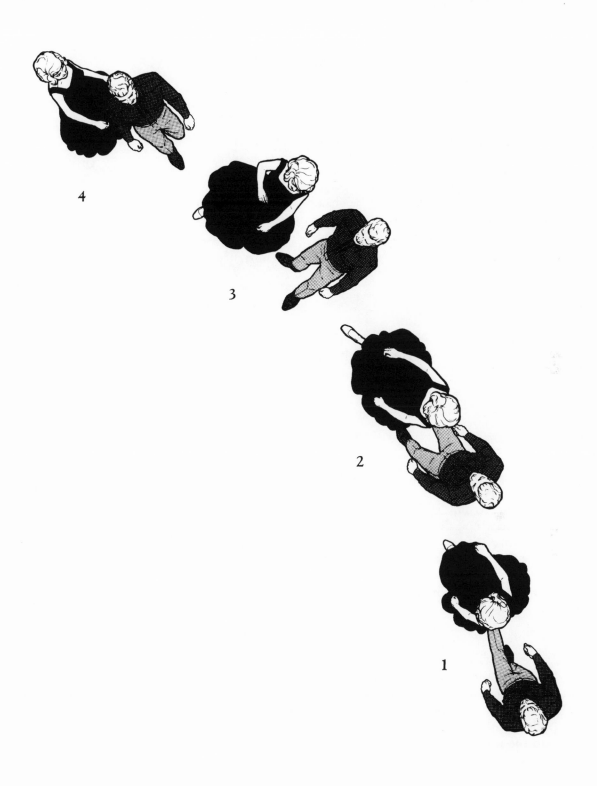

Figure 27.  Turnback

# Rollback

*To promenading dancers*

The call for this maneuver is "Roll back." It is delivered to dancers in rotary or circular formations. They may be either member, or both, within each couple in a Star Promenade or Couple Promenade (both described at their own entries further on).

*Also lone promenaders*

They also may be selected individual dancers, such as all the gents or all the ladies, or head gents, or the like, from among those promenading in single file around the ring.

*Like Turnback but different*

The movement executed by each dancer bears a very strong resemblance to a Turnback, but is not the same thing. For the dancer does not pivot sharply and return in the opposite direction along exactly the same path he just followed, as he does in a Turnback. Instead he makes a *very tight turn* to the right or the left, as appropriate.

*New path outside or inside*

Thus he enters a circular path just outside or—considerably less frequently—inside the one he previously followed. That is, a path slightly larger or smaller in diameter than the former one. He proceeds along this path in the direction opposite to that in which he moved before he turned.

*Couple roll back*

If both members of a couple in a Couple Promenade or a Star Promenade are instructed to roll back, each turns in his own direction. That is, the one on the outside rolls to the outside, and the one on the inside to the inside. In such circumstances some callers prefer to use more specific instructions, such as "Ladies roll out, gents roll in."

*To inside more like Turnback*

There is plenty of room on the outside of any circular or rotary formation for a dancer to roll outward. But there is precious little on the inside of, say, a Star Promenade, for a dancer to roll inward. Therefore, as a matter of practicality, a Rollback to the inside of such a formation has to be more like a Turnback than does a Rollback to the outside of the same formation.

*From single file*

Dancers promenading in single file roll out or in as directed, most commonly outward. To assure that the dancers understand what he expects them to do, a caller often will give them simplified instructions such as "Step out and turn back." In the absence of specific instructions, the dancers roll out.

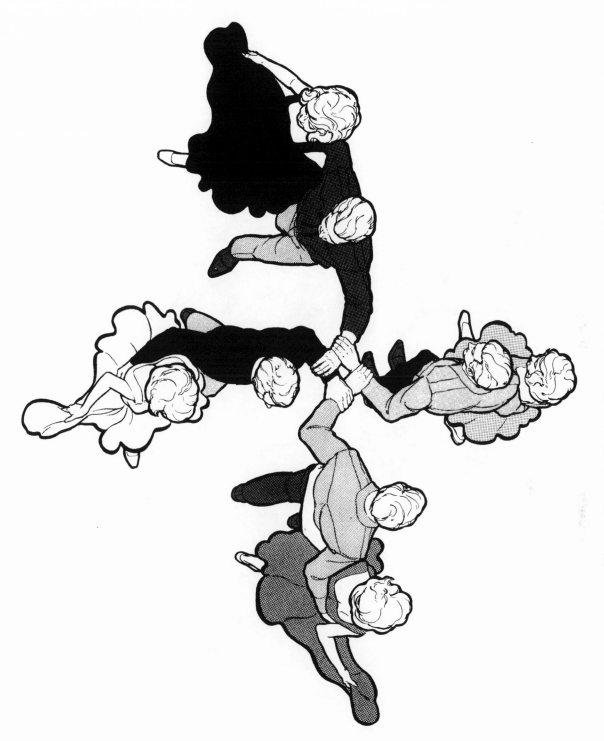

Figure 28. Rollback (Frame 1 in a sequence of 3)

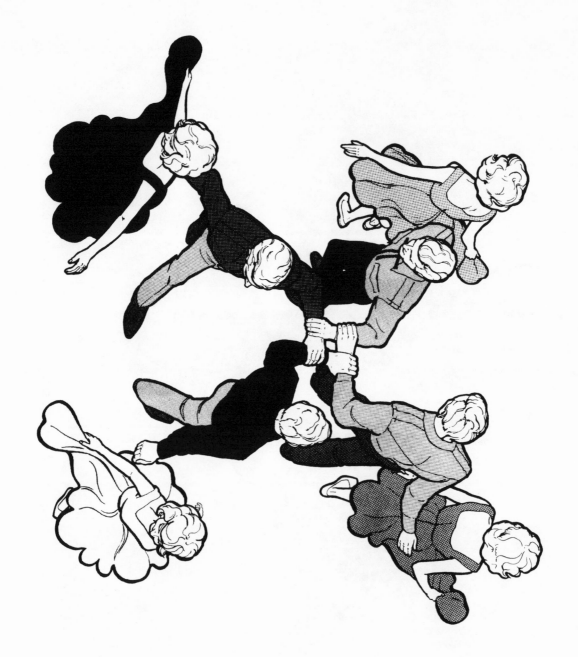

Figure 29. Rollback (Frame 2 in a sequence of 3)

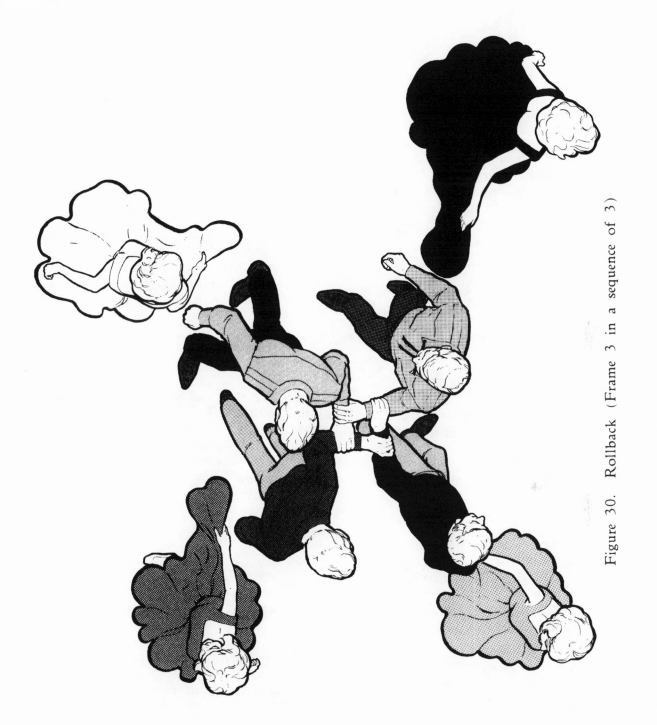

Figure 30. Rollback (Frame 3 in a sequence of 3)

# Weave the Ring

*Two columns opposite*

In executing this figure, two columns of dancers, each promenading in single file, move simultaneously around the same circular course in opposite directions. The gents move counterclockwise, the ladies clockwise.

*Move over to left*

As a given dancer approaches one person, each of them moves slightly to his left so as to give way on his right. Thus, without touching in any way, they pass right shoulder to right shoulder.

*Next move to right*

As the dancer approaches the next person, each of them moves slightly to his right so as to give way on his left. Thus, again without touching, those two pass left shoulder to left shoulder.

*Trace out weaving path*

The giving way alternately on the right and on the left by each dancer as he proceeds in the circular traffic pattern causes him to trace out a winding, weaving track interwoven with that of the dancers going the other way. Hence the name of the figure.

*Like Grand Right and Left*

This maneuver is exactly the same as the Grand Right and Left (described at its own entry further on), except that no Pullbys (also described later) are performed.

*Must remain alert*

Since the figures are so very much alike, and Grand Right and Left is the more common of the two, the dancer is almost certain to extend his hand to perform a Pullby if he has a momentary lapse of memory.

*Confusion results*

The person the hand is offered to is quite apt to take it, practically as an automatic response. Seeing this, others in the ring are influenced by the action and tempted to follow suit because of lack of confidence in their own memory. Thus mass confusion often ensues in short order from just one error by one dancer.

*Occupied hands prevent confusion*

To prevent the occurrence of this unhappy chain of events, each gent usually holds his hands in the small of his back, and each lady uses hers to work her skirt as she moves along. See the article on Promenade Alone, which appears earlier in this same functional group, for details concerning ways to hold the hands and arms while promenading in single file.

# Group 7. DIVIDING AND ENCIRCLING MOVEMENTS

## Split (or Divide) the Ring

*Forward and thru*

This could just as well have been called Split Your Opposites. The couples or individual dancers designated by the caller to be active move forward to the couple opposite them and pass between the members of that couple.

*Opposite couple move apart*

As the active dancers approach them, the members of the opposite couple drop hands and move apart a short step each to make it easy for the active dancers to get thru.

*Move together again*

As soon as the active dancers have passed between them, the members of the couple being split come together again. The next call tells the active dancers what to do after splitting the ring.

*May not look like ring*

The reader should note that the "ring" may not look much like a ring. Because it may (and in fact usually does) consist, in the main, of open space. That is, the members of the set do not have their hands joined so as to form a Circle.

*In home positions*

Rather, the four couples are standing in their home positions, with considerable space between them. But one must keep it in mind that if the dancers were to extend their arms and spread apart a bit, they would indeed form a ring.

## Split Corners

*Call to opposite couples*

The call for this maneuver always is directed to two opposite couples. Those couples move forward toward each other and meet in the center of the set. There each gent takes his opposite lady's left hand in his right, and they make a ¼ turn (90°) to the gent's left (the lady's right).

*Move to gent's corner*

They proceed side by side as a couple, the lady on the gent's right, to the gent's corner and split that couple.

## (Go) Round One (or Two, or Other Number)

*Supplementary instruction*

The call for this movement is issued as a supplementary instruction. Usually it follows a call such as "Split the ring" or "Cross trail." It tells an active dancer how many *persons* (NOT couples) he should go around.

*Halfway round unless*

If the caller does not mention the amount of encircling movement to be performed, it is understood he means halfway round (180°), so as to head back in the opposite direction. But he may specify any amount. The subsequent call tells the active dancers what to do next.

# Group 8. PASS THRU

*Facing lines*

This maneuver is performed by facing lines of dancers. Each line consists of either one or two couples. Four counts (beats of the music) are needed to execute the Pass Thru.

Each gent's partner is on his right. They walk beside each other, either holding nearest hands or without touching. The lines move toward each other.

*Gents move to left*

As the lines approach, each gent releases his partner's hand, if he has been holding it, and moves slightly to his left so as to give way on his right.

*Straight ahead or to left*

When lines containing only one couple each pass thru, each lady continues along the same path she started out on. And when two lines of four pass thru, the same holds true for the end ladies.

But the lady in the middle of each line of four has to give way on her right by moving to her left enough to provide room for the middle gents to get thru without colliding with each other, or one of them with her.

*No touching*

Each dancer and the person he meets pass right shoulder to right shoulder *without touching*. While staying abreast of his partner, each gent immediately veers back to his right enough to reestablish the proper distance between his partner and him and align himself directly behind the back of the lady he just passed by on the left of.

*Halt if no more calls*

After passing thru the other line and reaching the position just vacated by it, each line halts in place if further instructions have not been given. The members are still facing out of the square, either at right angles or some lesser angle to a side of it, their backs to the line they just passed thru.

*Two can pass thru*

Two individual dancers can pass thru, although they seldom do. But if, for example, there are two facing lines, the call "Ends pass thru" can be given.

In such an event, the two facing dancers at each double end of the pairs of lines come toward each other, move slightly to their left so as to give way on their right, and pass by each other right shoulder to right shoulder.

*May not seem like thru*

Offhand, it may not seem that two real lines pass *thru* each other in this situation. It might appear that each "line" consists of only one dancer (an end person in the original line) and, therefore, that the two of them pass *around*, or *by*, but not *thru*, each other.

Such is not the case, however. It is accurate to say that each line is only a partial line, a portion of the original one. But it still is a real line, because it consists of *both* end dancers, not just one of them.

*Do actually pass thru*

Being at each end of the complete line, the two dancers are rather widely separated. Nevertheless, as they move along parallel with each other toward the fragment of the other line, they do still constitute a line. Hence each of these lines, with a great gap in its middle, truly passes *thru* the other.

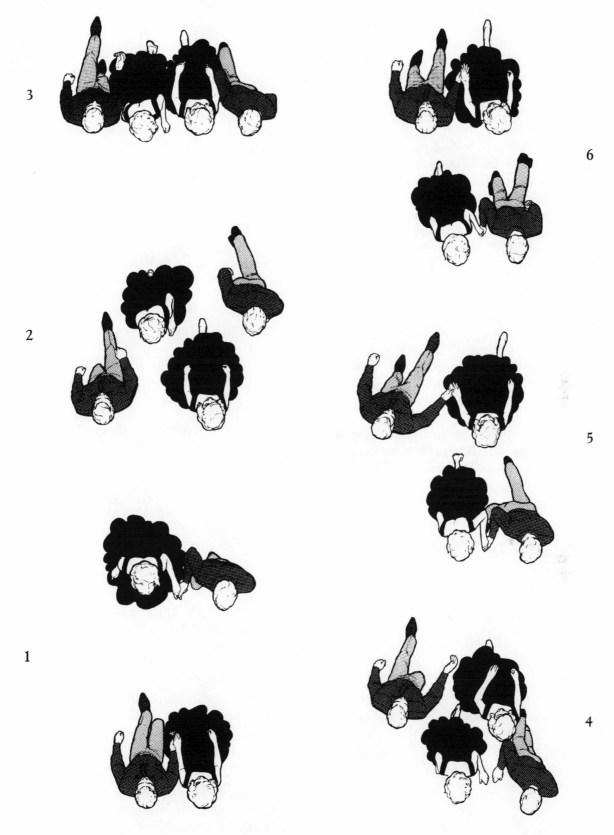

Figure 31.  Pass Thru

47

# Group 9. CROSS TRAIL

This maneuver is performed by lines. They can either be isolated or facing each other. Facing ones first execute a Pass Thru before each of them separately enters the Cross Trail proper.

Far most commonly a line consists of just one couple. Therefore a couple will be used in the description of the maneuver to be given here.

*Takes four counts*

Whether performed by isolated or facing couples, the Cross Trail itself (proper) requires four counts (beats of the music) to execute.

*Lady to left*

As the members of an isolated couple progress beside each other, the lady veers to the left and crosses in front of the gent. That is, farther along than him in their general line of travel.

*Gent to right*

Taking a step slightly shorter than usual, the gent slows enough to allow his partner to cross ahead of him as he veers to the right and passes behind her. That is, not so far along as her in their general line of travel.

*Catches up, veers back*

Then he takes a couple of longer steps to increase his speed and come abreast of her again, on her right. As he does so, he veers back to the left very slightly—enough to make his path once again parallel with hers and space himself the proper distance from her.

*Lady's movements*

The lady's movements are practically a mirror image of the gent's. She veers first to her left, as she crosses over, then very

slightly to her right, to make her path again parallel with the gent's. As he is catching up with her on her right side she slows slightly to make it easier for him to overtake her.

*Facing pass thru first*

When this maneuver is performed by facing, rather than isolated couples, they first perform a Pass Thru. As soon as the members of each couple have passed beyond the other couple, they enter the Cross Trail proper.

*Has to be more nimble*

When facing couples execute Cross Trail, the gent in each of them has to be more nimble than when he is a member of an isolated couple performing the maneuver.

*Is displaced to left*

The reason is that although the lady in each couple can (and should) go almost straight ahead during the Pass Thru, the gent is displaced to the left by that maneuver.

*Lady can't veer too much*

After they are thru the Pass Thru, the lady still can veer to the left only the normal amount. For if she veers more, she displaces their twin paths to the left of where they ought to be.

Thus to cross over behind her after the Pass Thru and get to her right side in the Cross Trail, the gent has to travel almost twice as far as usual.

*Should slow longer*

Therefore the lady should slow down a bit longer than she would in an isolated Cross Trail. That enables the gent to reach her right side in the same length of time he would take in the isolated Cross Trail.

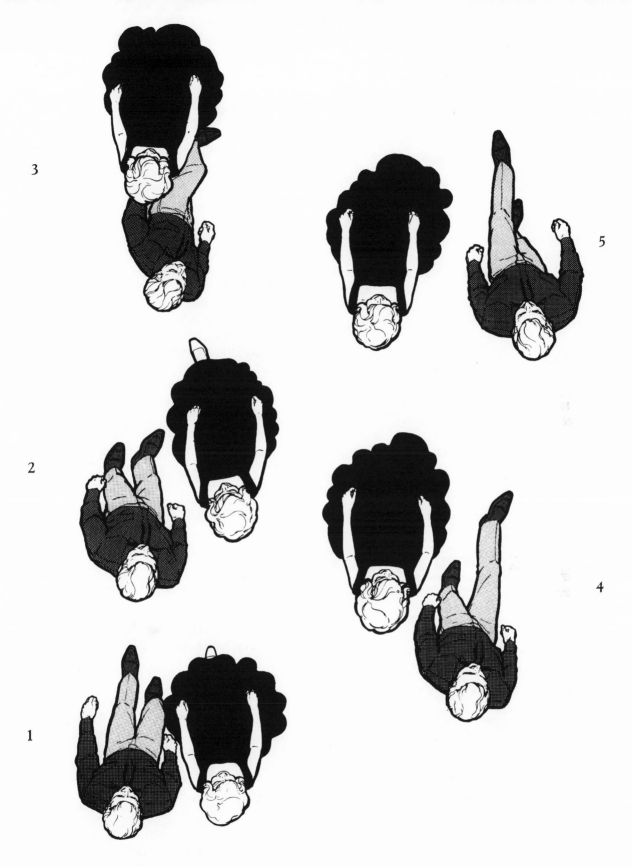

Figure 32.    Cross Trail

49

# Group 10. PULLBY MANEUVERS

## Pullby

*No noun title until now*

The expression "Pull her (on) by" has been used for years as a *call*. But until now there has been no noun title for the movement itself. The name Pullby is one devised by the author for convenience in referring to the maneuver.

*Lines of dancers*

The movement can be performed by any number of dancers arranged in two lines of even numbers. But often each line consists of only one dancer. That is, often only two dancers participate.

*Counts needed*

Two counts (beats of the music) are required to execute the Pullby.

*Don't be rough*

The dancer must be scrupulously careful not to jerk or yank on the other's hand, or to squeeze it excessively, in pulling by. The gents in particular have to guard against this, for they have more tendency toward roughness than the ladies do. The movement should always be executed with gentle grace, light and smooth thruout.

# Righthand Pullby

*Move to left*

The dancers approach head on. Each moves slightly to his left, so as to give way on his right, as in a Pass Thru. But he does not merely pass on by without touching the other person. Instead, each dancer extends his right arm straight out, at about the waist level of the gent, and takes the other's right hand.

*Grasp like handshake*

Hands are clasped exactly as in a handshake, but only for a short time and with no more force than absolutely necessary. They remain in the same position in space, above the dance floor, as the dancers move toward each other.

*Hands fixed in position*

To achieve this temporary fixity of the hands, each dancer allows his arm to bend at the elbow more and more as he approaches the other person.

*Arms straighten out*

As the two draw abreast and pass on by each other one step, right shoulder to right shoulder, each allows his arm to straighten out again. When the pair have taken one step past each other and no longer can maintain the grip, they release hands.

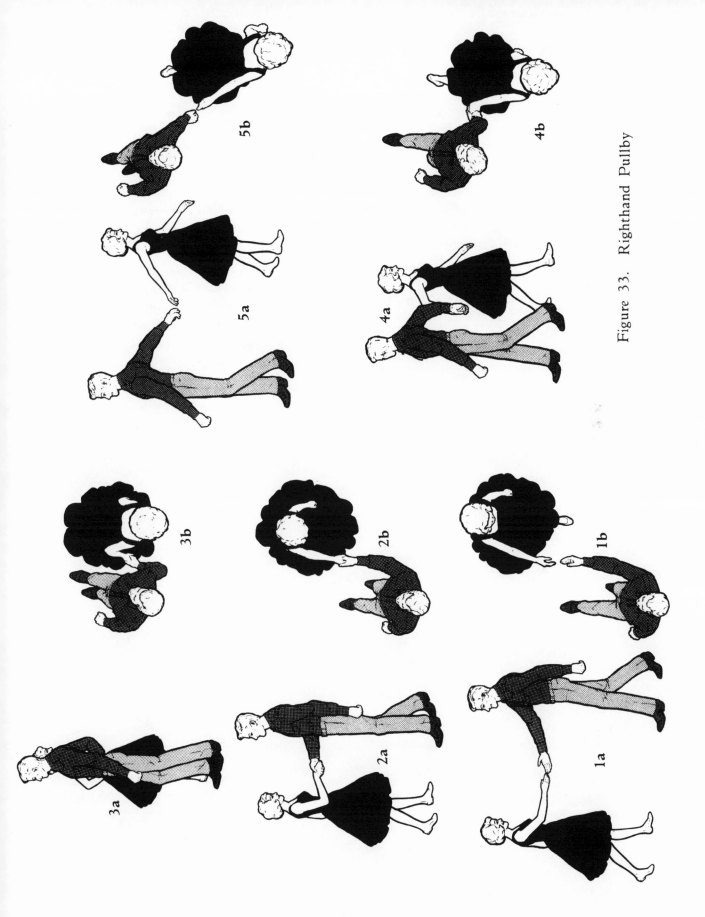

Figure 33. Righthand Pullby

51

# Lefthand Pullby

*Opposite of Righthand Pullby*

This is a mirror image of the Righthand Pullby. That is, everything in that maneuver is reversed, right to left.

*Move to right*

Each dancer moves slightly to his right so as to give way on his left, clasps the other's left hand in his left, and pulls by, breaking the handclasp after the two have taken one step past each other.

*Don't be rough*

The same precautions must be taken into consideration in executing this maneuver as are observed in performing a Righthand Pullby. That is, the dancer must be scrupulously careful not to jerk or yank on the other dancer's hand, or to squeeze it excessively, in pulling by. He should strive for a light, smooth look and feel thruout the movement.

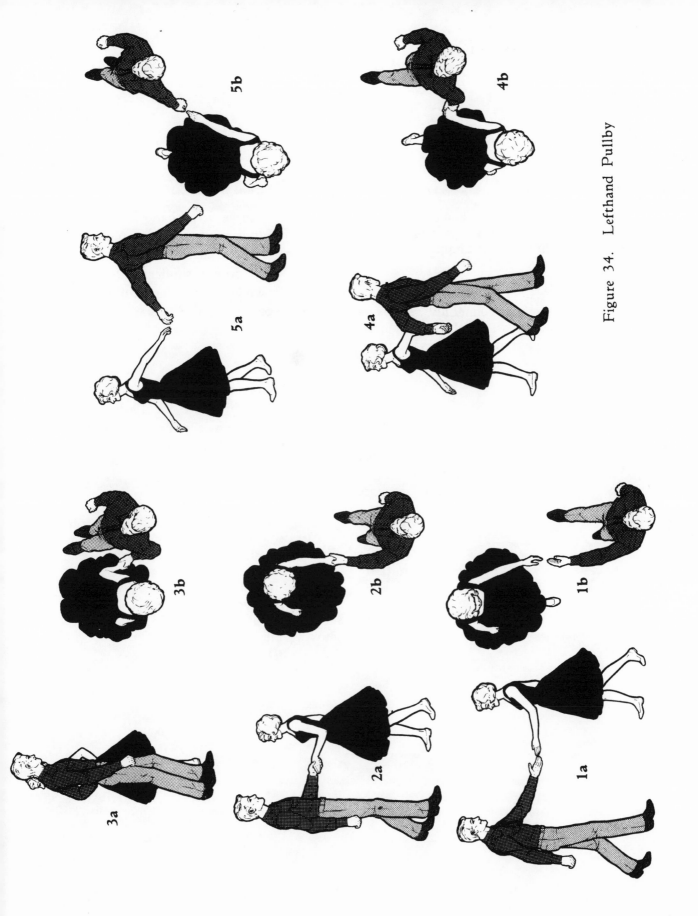

Figure 34. Lefthand Pullby

# Grand Right and Left

*Other name*

Another name for this maneuver, used where it rhymes better with some particular word, is Right and Left Grand.

*Often follows, not always*

This figure very commonly follows an Allemande Left (described further along in the book); but it does not have to. It can be entered in a number of other ways.

*Gents one way, ladies other*

However it is entered, it begins with all the gents facing counterclockwise (as viewed from above), and all the ladies clockwise, around the circle thought of as superimposed within the basic reference square.

*Righthand Pullby with partner*

The lady that any given gent initially faces is her partner. They execute a Righthand Pullby. Then the gent continues moving in his direction around the ring and his partner in hers.

*Lefthand Pullby with next, etc*

He performs a Lefthand Pullby with the next lady he meets, a Righthand Pullby with the one after that, etc. Meanwhile his partner is performing similar Pullbys with the gents while moving around the ring in the opposite direction.

*Fifth person met is partner*

Therefore the fifth person any dancer encounters is his partner. They always meet again in the position opposite the position they started from.

*Usually promenade back home*

When they meet, they may be instructed to do any one of a number of things. But far most usually—customarily—they promenade back home. If they do, they proceed in the normal direction for a Couple Promenade (described later in the book), which is the way the gent has been moving all along.

## Square Thru

*Move around small square*

This figure derives its name from the path traversed by the dancers performing it. Two gents move clockwise, and two ladies counterclockwise, in a square pattern.

*Smaller than basic one*

The square they trace out as they move is much smaller than the basic reference square. It is only about three feet on a side—the length needed for a dancer to take two ordinary shuffle steps. It can lie almost anywhere within or around the ba-sic square, depending upon where the maneuver is begun.

*Two couples face*

The two couples face. Thruout this figure, each dancer's opposite is the member of the other couple who faces him as the maneuver begins. His partner is of course the person who initially stands beside him.

*Gents right first, ladies left*

THE FOLLOWING HOLDS TRUE FOR EITHER RIGHT OR LEFT SQUARE THRU:

*A gent should lead off with his* RIGHT *foot, a lady with her* LEFT.

# Right (Ordinary) Square Thru

*"One" as first released*

Leading off with his right foot, the gent performs a Righthand Pullby with his opposite lady. Both of them should consciously and deliberately make a mental note of "One" (meaning "One pullby performed," or "One hand passed") as they release hands.

*Should not linger*

The dancer should not prolong the grip on any hand he passes. That is, he should not delay releasing hands, but should "break clean," as a referee tells the boxers to do.

*Must keep count thruout*

It is very important that all dancers in the Square Thru keep accurate count of the number of hands they have passed if the call, which can have several explicit forms, is to be properly followed.

*Gent sharp turn to right*

The gent takes one step beyond his opposite lady, then makes a sharp, abrupt 90° pivot (¼ turn in place) to the right on the ball of his left foot, stepping off smartly on his right foot as he begins a Lefthand Pullby with his partner.

*Lady sharp turn to left*

The ladies use the same hands as the gents, but pivot to the *left* on the ball of their *right* foot each time, so as to proceed counterclockwise in the square pattern. Everyone should take care to make rapid, sharp pivots at true right angles and avoid slow, sloppy turns at other angles.

*As released, not before*

Also, each dancer should be sure to tick off the total number of hands passed as each hand is *released*, not as it is grasped or before. It would not seem that it would matter much whether one counts the hands as he takes them or as he releases them, but it can definitely make a difference.

*Effect of counting prematurely*

For there is a tendency to count the last hand in anticipation, before taking it, then fail to actually take it before attempting to go into the next maneuver. If he does this, the dancer is liable to position himself in such a way as to make it difficult, or perhaps completely impossible, to enter that maneuver properly.

*Thru number specified*

The four dancers squaring thru proceed as described above, each gent performing alternate Righthand and Lefthand Pullbys with his opposite lady and his partner, respectively, for the number of hands specified or indicated by the call.

*Number of hands varies*

For the explicit forms of the figure consist in the number of hands called for. It might, for instance, be for only "One hand round" (or "One hand thru"), which is Quarter Square Thru. But this form is rare.

*Other numbers of hands*

Or it might be for Half Square Thru (two hands round), which is quite common. Threequarter Square Thru (three hands round) is even more often met with. But Full Square Thru (four hands round) is probably the most prevalent of all. The caller usually allots ten counts (beats of the music) for it to be performed.

*More than four hands*

It is by no means uncommon for even more than four hands to be called for. If so, the dancers simply repeat the procedure described above thru the appropriate number of additional hands.

*No pivot after last Pullby*

THE DANCER MUST REMEMBER that as he completes the last Pullby of the Square Thru, *he does* NOT *pivot.* Therefore *he always ends up back to back* with the last person he pulled by, ready to follow the next call.

*Beginner's tendency*

The beginner often has a strong tendency to do the following. He takes the last hand for the final Pullby, all right. But then he fails to do what he should do after that: Pull on by, drop the hand, and go into the next maneuver.

Instead he holds onto the hand and, in the desperation born of confusion, attempts to perform some completely different maneuver (instead of the one called) with *that* person.

*Unvarying rule*

IT IS IMPORTANT TO REMEMBER that *a dancer always performs the next maneuver with a person who is* NOT *one of the three with whom he executed the Square Thru.*

# Left Square Thru

*Less common*

This figure is considerably less common than the ordinary (Right) Square Thru, but it is not remarkably unusual. It too can be called for any number of hands round.

*Not mirror image*

*It is* NOT *a mirror image of a regular Square Thru*. The flows of traffic in the square pattern are the same in both figures: Gents clockwise, ladies counterclockwise.

*Differs in only one way*

The Left Square Thru differs from the regular Square Thru in only one small way: *It is begun with a* LEFTHAND *Pullby instead of a Righthand Pullby.*

*Start with same feet*

The dancer moves in the same direction as in a regular Square Thru. Accordingly, HE SHOULD LEAD OFF WITH THE SAME FOOT HE DOES IN A REGULAR SQUARE THRU: a gent with the right, a lady with the left.

# Group 11.   ARM SWINGS

The term Arm Swings is the designation given to a class of swings in which contact between dancers is limited to the arm or some part of it, such as the hand.

In the Forearm Swing there is contact along all or part of the forearm, and the hand grasps either the elbow joint or the forearm below it. Thus we have the Forearm Swing with either elbow grip or forearm grip.

In addition, there is another type of arm swing in which contact is limited to the hand. It is called, appropriately enough, the Hand Swing.

Therefore these swings fall into the following categories.

## Arm Swings

a. Forearm Swing

   1. With Elbow Grip

   2. With Forearm Grip

b. Hand Swing

Not too long ago, there was very little uniformity in usage of these terms. Even now, unfortunately, standardization is not complete, and there is still some confusion in names.

For instance, the Forearm Swing, although actually a division of the general class called Arm Swings, is itself sometimes referred as an "arm swing."

Occasionally, also, the Forearm Swing is referred to as a "righthand" or "lefthand" swing. Even more confusingly, the Forearm Swing now and then is called a "righthand" or "lefthand" *turn*. Fortunately, this usage is becoming less prevalent.

Hopefully, standardization will improve as time goes on. The present disorder in terms does not usually bother the experienced dancer too much, but on occasion can cause even him some trouble. And it certainly is confusing—and discouraging—to the beginner. Hence the detailed explanation given here.

# Forearm Swing

## With Elbow Grip

*Dancers face*

Two dancers face each other. Each extends the same arm (right or left, as appropriate) in front of him, the elbow bent and the forearm roughly horizontal.

*Hands grasp joints*

The forearms are parallel, touching along their inside surfaces, and each hand grasps the other person's elbow joint. The open palm of the hand is against the inside of the other's elbow joint, and the thumb is on the outside of the joint.

*Below gent's joint*

Gents' arms generally are a little longer than ladies'. Therefore when the gent grips the lady's elbow joint with his hand, her hand usually will be very slightly below his elbow joint. But it will not be far enough from it to impair the hold appreciably.

*Positive, secure grip*

The elbow grip is by its nature a very secure hold, and it is made even more positive by the contact of the parallel forearms. For this reason, very little hand grip is

necessary. Whatever pressure is employed should be exerted evenly, by the whole hand. The dancer ought to be careful not to apply most of the force with the thumb, and thus dig it into the other's arm.

*Can walk, should swing*

After the hold is established, the dancers can simply walk around each other in the appropriate direction, moving in a lively manner. But for a really good swing, though, they should not just walk around, but dynamically (though smoothly) *swing* around.

*For best feel*

That is, they should "give each other some resistance" by leaning away from each other slightly, as they should do in any swing. Doing so causes the swing to have a much more satisfying feel to it.

*Turn appropriate amount*

They turn around an amount determined by the circumstances, but far most often halfway round (180°). For that amount of turning, four counts (beats of the music) usually are allotted.

*Open Spacing*

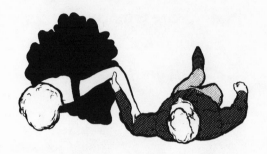

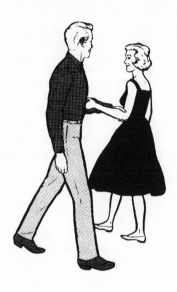 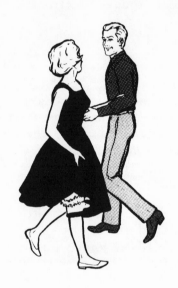

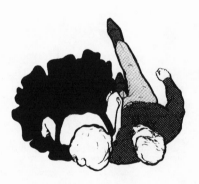

*Close Spacing*

Figure 35.   (Left) Forearm Swing with Elbow Grip

60

## With Forearm Grip

*Above wrist, below elbow*

In some areas of the country it is customary to grasp just above the wrist. In other areas it is standard practice to grasp farther up, but still below the elbow. The exact distance up the forearm varies not only from area to area, but from group to group within a given area.

*Many use it*

The forearm grip for the Forearm Swing is one that thousands of dancers find perfectly satisfactory and use all the time. And it is not the purpose of this book to mount a campaign to do away with this useful, serviceable hold. Nonetheless, one thing should be pointed out.

*Does have shortcomings*

It is an indisputable fact of human anatomy that the forearm has a tapering cross section. It follows, therefore, that gripping anywhere between elbow and wrist simply has to require more pressure, for a positive grasp, than does a hold on the elbow joint. Thus it can be seen that the forearm grip is inherently less secure, less comfortable, and less dependable than the elbow grip.

*Counts allotted*

Four counts (beats of the music) are usually allowed for turning halfway round (180°) in the Forearm Swing with a forearm grip, just as with the elbow grip.

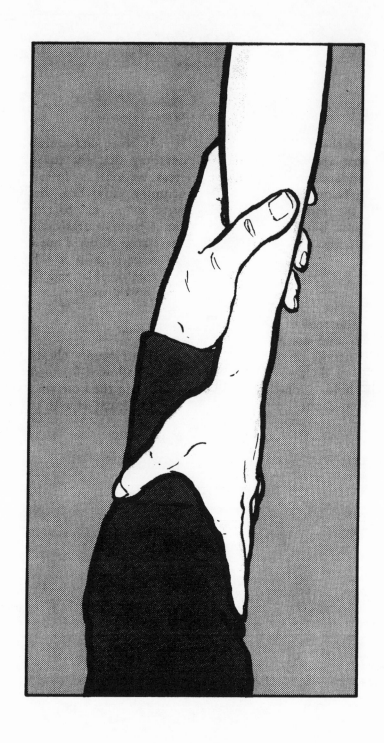

Figure 36.  Forearm Grip for  (Left)  Forearm Swing

# Hand Swing

*Sometimes called "turn"*

The Hand Swing, more commonly than the Forearm Swing or any other swing, is occasionally called a "turn." But use of the word *turn*, even in this application, is declining more and more as time goes on.

*Form of Forearm Swing*

The Hand Swing and the Forearm Swing are virtually the same thing in slightly different forms. They are used for the same purpose, and they are performed in the same manner.

*Difference*

The only difference is that in the Forearm Swing the pair grasp each other's elbow joint or forearm, while in the Hand Swing they grasp hands exactly as in shaking hands, but with only enough grip to ensure a firm hold.

*Can walk, should swing*

After the handclasp is established, the dancers can simply walk around each other in the appropriate direction, moving in a lively manner. For a really good swing, though, they should not just walk around,

but dynamically (though smoothly) *swing* around.

*For best feel*

That is, they should "give each other some resistance" by leaning away from each other slightly, as they should in any swing. Doing so causes the swing to have a much more satisfying feel to it.

*Slower; needs more room*

Because the arms are extended during a Hand Swing, it requires more room than the Forearm Swing does. Also, because the dancers must move farther, it is not as fast as the Forearm Swing. Therefore the Hand Swing is appropriate for relatively open, slow-moving squares, while the Forearm Swing (particularly with an elbow grip) is well suited to compact, fast-moving sets.

*Not as firm, but satisfactory*

The hold in the Hand Swing is not quite as firm and steady as the elbow grip that can be employed in the Forearm Swing, but in general it is equally satisfactory. And in several maneuvers a Hand Swing has to be employed; a Forearm Swing is not suitable.

# 11. ARM SWINGS

## CHOICE OF FOREARM OR HAND SWING

*Depends on several things*

Which of the two swings is used depends not only upon the area and the club, but also the individual himself. Each gent has full freedom to decide for himself, each time an arm swing is in order, whether he will use a Forearm Swing or a Hand Swing.

*May choose either*

Depending upon the condition of the specific figure in progress, the circumstances of the moment, or perhaps nothing more than his own fancy, he may decide to perform a Forearm Swing.

*May later choose other*

A minute later he may choose to use the Hand Swing. And at present he will not be frowned upon for using either one of them in preference to the other in either instance. Nor will he be considered inconsistent for using first one, then the other.

*Counts allotted*

Six counts (beats of the music) are generally considered necessary for the dancer to complete a Hand Swing halfway round (180°).

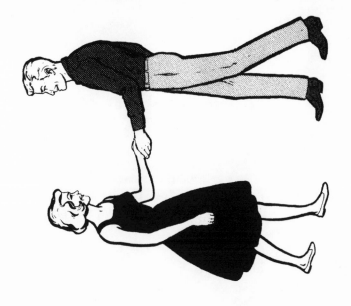

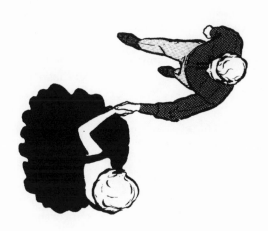

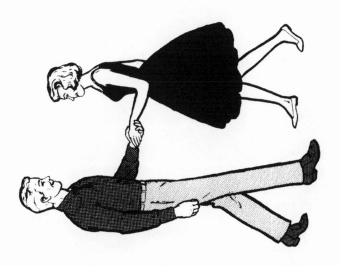

Figure 37. (Left) Hand Swing

65

# Allemande Left

*Even nondancers know*

Because this is one of the oldest maneuvers in squaredancing, its name is known even to many who do not squaredance. For this reason, beginners often expect it to be especially fancy, or particularly difficult, or remarkable in some other way.

*Nothing fancy*

But the actual fact of the matter is that it now is nothing more than a plain, unglamorous Left Forearm (or Left Hand) Swing performed with a particular person: one's corner.

*Executed with corner*

True, it is not an Allemande Left unless it is performed with one's corner. But in execution it is identical in every respect with any other Left Forearm (or Hand) Swing. (We are ignoring here one particular way of executing it that is a refinement not suited to a beginner's course.)

*Most-performed maneuver*

Nevertheless, its fame is deserved. The Allemande Left is not glamorous, but it is the veritable backbone of squaredancing, and the dancer probably will perform it more often than any other maneuver.

*Even best sometimes goof*

It is all too easy to become discombooberated by the intricacies of some grabbag figure or other that one needs to file a flight plan to execute. Even the seasoned veterans are thrown for a loss occasionally.

*Wedge to get back in*

When that happens, however, the dancer has one recourse he can always rely on. He knows he can wait for the welcome call for a good old Allemande Left and start in again at that point.

Regardless of how mixed up he may have become, the *knows* that he knows how to perform the tried and true Allemande Left. Thus it acts as a "wedge" to get him back into the action.

*Variant name*

Left Allemande is merely a variant name, sometimes used where it is more suitable for rhyming with some particular word, for this same maneuver.

# Group 12. WAIST SWING

*Plain "swing" means this*

The plain word "swing," without a descriptive adjective, practically always means a Waist Swing. The call to "Swing your partner (or corner, or some other lady)" always tells the dancers to execute this movement.

*Stance like ballroom*

The gent and the lady assume a stance quite like that for regular ballroom dancing. But instead of being face to face, they are very nearly right hip to right hip.

*Positions of hands*

The gent holds the lady's right hand in his left at about the level of her shoulder and puts his right arm around her waist, holding his right hand firmly in the small of her back.

She places her left hand either on his right shoulder or on his right arm just below the shoulder. She does not put her arm around his neck, as she might in ballroom dancing.

*Move clockwise*

The pair should stay loose and relaxed, and not hold each other too closely. They begin to move forward around each other to the right (clockwise, as viewed from above) in the following way.

*Push with left, pivot around right*

Each of them puts his right foot forward so that the outsides of those feet almost touch. Each keeps the ball of his right foot fixed in position, temporarily, and pivots around it during each push with the left foot.

*Most of weight on right*

The right foot supports most of the weight, but part of it is shifted momentarily to the left toes each time the left foot is brought round, in a short step, one third or so of the small clockwise circle it traces out.

*Left always to left of right*

The left foot always is to the left of the right foot in the direction of turning. At the beginning of one push, the left toes are about 12 inches to the left of a line lengthwise thru the middle of the right foot and four or five inches in front of a crosswise line thru the right toes. At this time the right heel is lifted slightly (about 1/2 inch).

*Like scooter, but rotary*

The action is that of a child on a scooter, except that the push from the left toes is used to turn the body in a rotary motion instead of moving it along a straight line.

*Foot positions after push*

At the completion of the push, the left toes still are about 12 inches to the left of the right foot, but now are either even with a crosswise line thru the right heel or two or three inches behind such a line. The right heel can be dropped lightly to the floor as the left foot is moved round into position for the next push.

*Traces tiny circle*

As mentioned previously, each dancer pivots about the ball of his right foot dur-

## 12. Waist Swing

ing each push with the left. However, at the completion of each push with the left, the right is advanced just a few inches forward and to the right around another—even smaller—clockwise circle that is not much larger in diameter than the length of the foot itself.

*Between right feet*

Although each of the dancers repeatedly pivots momentarily about his right foot, the pair as a unit rotate about a central pivot point between the two right feet. For a good swing, the pair should lean away from each other slightly, as they should in any swing.

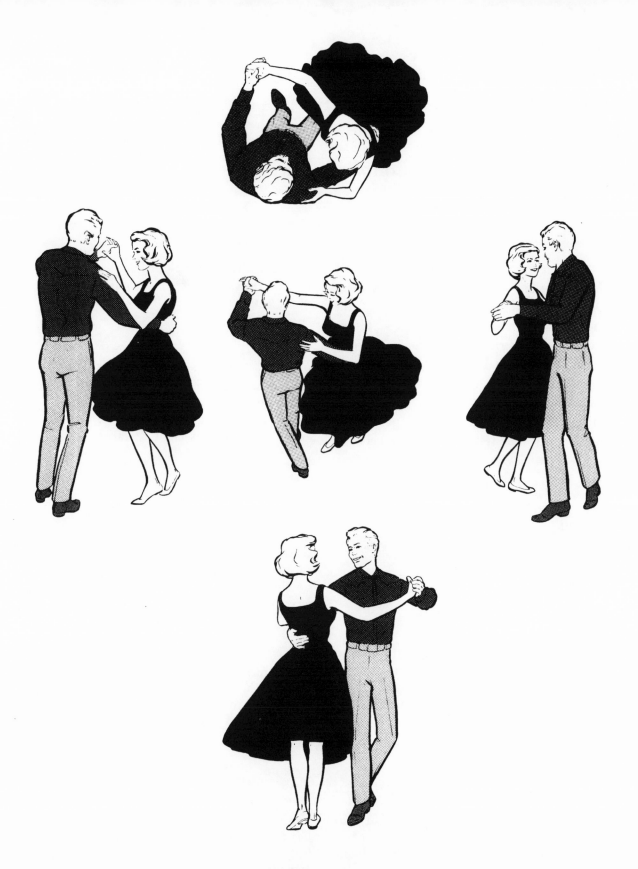

Figure 38.   Waist Swing

# Group 13.   TRAVEL AS A COUPLE

## Couple Promenade

*Several, this standard*

There are several combinations of hand positions and holds that can be used. One is popular in a certain section of the country and another one elsewhere. However, the one described here is the most widespread, and it can be considered the standard stance. Its prevalence probably is accounted for by the fact that it is simple and unaffected. Its naturalness gives it a very comfortable feel for both partners.

*Side by side, gent on left*

The gent and his partner face in the same direction and stand side by side, the gent on the left.

*Gent's left hand in front of right hip*

He extends his left arm horizontally, just above waist level, rather sharply across his body so that his left hand, palm up, is eight or ten inches in front of his right hip.

*Right forearm ahead, slightly to right*

His right forearm also is horizontal and just above waist level. He positions his right elbow directly above his right hip and extends his right forearm forward—not directly along a line straight out in front of the hip, but very slightly to the right.

*Right hand, left hand*

Thus the gent's right hand is level with his left one, eight or ten inches to the right of it, and a few inches forward of it.

*Left on left, right on right*

The lady extends her arms and bends her elbows the proper amount to place her hands, palms down, on the gent's hands— left on left and right on right. Her left forearm goes under his right forearm.

*Close but not too close*

Holding her hands as described, the gent leads his partner ahead. Using the normal squaredance shuffle step, they move forward side by side. They should be close enough together to be comfortable, but not so close as to interfere with each other's movements in walking.

*Usually move to right*

Unless otherwise instructed, they move off to their right (counterclockwise, as viewed from above) around the circle thought of as superimposed within the basic reference square.

*Seldom less than halfway*

They either come back to the gent's home position (which they usually have left from) or stop in some other spot specified by the caller. He seldom has them promenade less than halfway round the ring, but may have them make 1½ circuits.

70

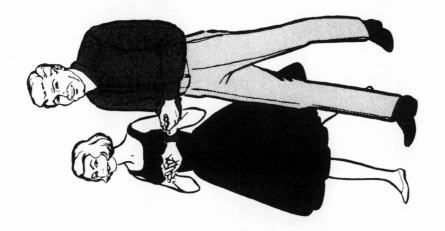

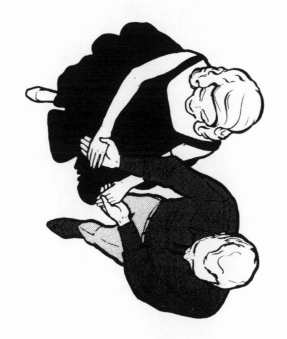

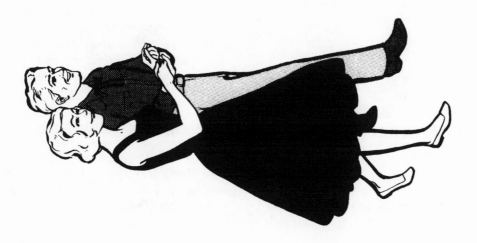

Figure 39.  Couple Promenade

71

# Wheelaround

*Gent stays on left*

By means of this maneuver, a promenading couple — acting as a unit — reverse their direction of travel, each member retaining his same position relative to the other. That is, the gent remains the left-hand member thruout.

*Counts allotted*

Three or four counts (beats of the music) are needed to perform the Wheelaround.

*Wheel to left*

Normal handholds for Couple Promenade are retained thruout the movement. The couple practically always wheel to the left, but on very rare occasions must wheel to the right. The usual case is described here.

*Gent is pivot*

Since they wheel to the left, the gent is the inside partner in the wheeling action —the one who acts as a pivot (but a moving pivot) as they whirl.

*One backward step forward*

He halts on his left foot and, as he pivots to the left on it, takes one step *backward*. The backward step is to the *right* and *forward* in the original direction of travel.

*Pivot on left, then right*

The pivoting on the left foot is merely momentary. It lasts only long enough

for him to take his backward step to the right and farther along. As soon as the right foot is brought down, *it* becomes the pivot for the remainder of the gent's turning action.

*Off from right in new direction*

As he is completing his ½ (180°) leftface turn, he swings his left foot about 18 inches directly to the left of its former position. Thus it is to the left of his right foot as he starts off from his right foot in the new direction.

*Lady tight left turn*

The gent must take his backward step slowly enough to avoid interfering with his partner as she walks on in a very tight turn to the left around him. She faces forward (in relation to her instantaneous direction of motion) thruout her turn.

*Move forward out of wheel*

As soon as the wheeling has been completed, the gent begins to move forward in the new direction, and the lady, who emerges from the wheeling facing in the new direction, continues moving forward that way.

*Opposite direction and paths*

After wheeling, the couple should move along exectly the same two-track course as they did before, but in the opposite direction. The gent should be on the lady's former path, and she on his. The

## Wheelaround

procedure described above displaces each the proper amount to align them as they should be.

### Gent must back up

It is essential the gent back up one step as described. If he just makes a tight turn similar to the lady's, or simply pivots in place without taking the step backward, the figure will not work out as it should.

### Paths will be offset

The two paths (his before reversing direction and hers afterward, and vice versa) will be offset from each other by at least the distance between the members of the couple while in the promenade stance.

### To individuals poor practice

Although it is not considered good practice, some callers do occasionally address the call for this maneuver to individual dancers. In such an event, the dancer should execute a Turnback.

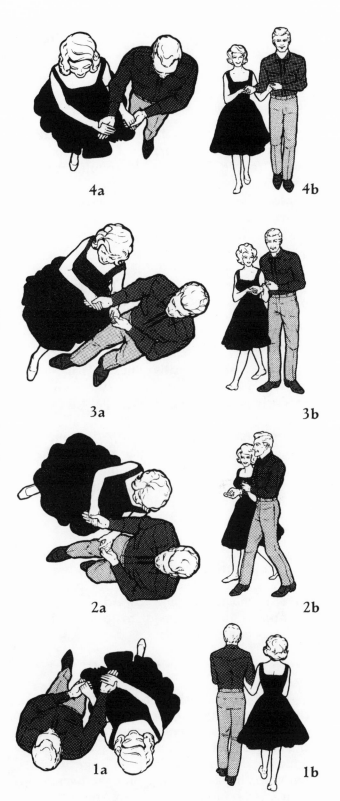

Figure 40.    Wheelaround

# Backtrack

*Gent becomes righthand member*

Thruout a Wheelaround, the gent remains the lefthand member of the promenading couple. But when the couple reverse direction of motion by executing a Backtrack, the gent changes from lefthand to righthand member.

*Counts allotted*

Two or three counts (beats of the music) are needed to complete the Backtrack.

*Several times in a row*

It is not especially unusual for this movement to be performed several times in fairly rapid succession. Whether that occurs or not, however, the Backtrack always commences, the first time, with the couple promenading in the normal manner, the gent on the left and the lady on the right. Her right and left hands rest, palms down, on his right and left hands, respectively.

*Virtually Turnbacks by both*

In executing the Backtrack, each member of the couple performs what amounts to a Turnback, turning toward the other member. Thus the gent turns to his right, and the lady to her left.

*Loose handholds*

They retain their handholds while they turn, but the grasp of the hands must, of necessity, vary considerably during the change from one direction of travel to the opposite. Holds must be kept quite loose while the hands are being brought over to their new positions, which are completely different from the original ones.

*Hand positions reversed*

When the couple promenade in the usual manner, holding their joined hands in front of them, their hands are near the gent's right hip and the lady's left hip. When the Backtrack is completed, the hands are near the gent's left hip and the lady's right hip.

*Gent's left ahead and·to left*

Now the gent's left hand is *ahead* of his right hand five or six inches and about the same distance to the *left* of it. His right hand still is at about the same level as his left, and the lady's hands still rest palms down on his.

*Forearm was under, now over*

But whereas her left forearm formerly went under his right forearm, now her *right* forearm goes *over* his *left* forearm. The gent now is the righthand member of the couple as they proceed in the new direction.

*Second one mirror image*

As mentioned previously, the call for a Backtrack may be given again while the couple are promenading with the gent on the right, their hands in the positions described. If so, the members simply perform a mirror image of the action described above.

*Revert to normal Promenade*

The gent turns to his left and the lady to her right, the two of them shifting their joined hands into the positions appropriate for an ordinary Couple Promenade. Thus they again promenade in the original direction in the normal manner, the gent once more the lefthand member of the couple.

*To individuals poor practice*

Although it is not considered good practice, some callers do occasionally address the call for this maneuver to individual dancers. In such an event, the dancer should execute a Turnback.

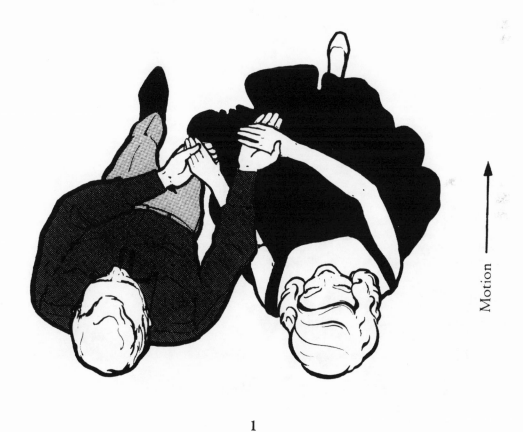

Motion

1

Figure 41.   Backtrack (Frame 1 in a sequence of 5)

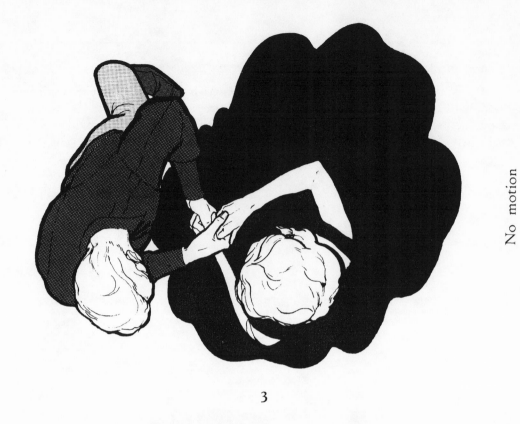

No motion

3

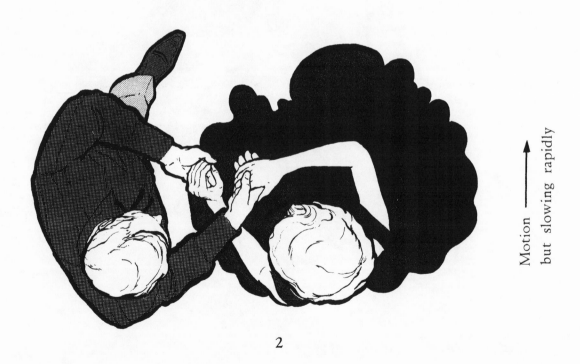

Motion →
but slowing rapidly

2

Figure 42.   Backtrack (Frames 2 and 3 in a sequence of 5)

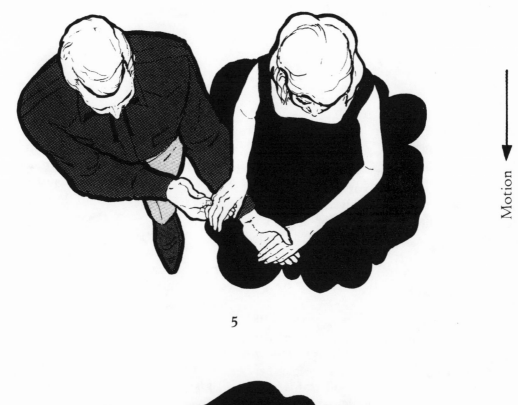

Motion

5

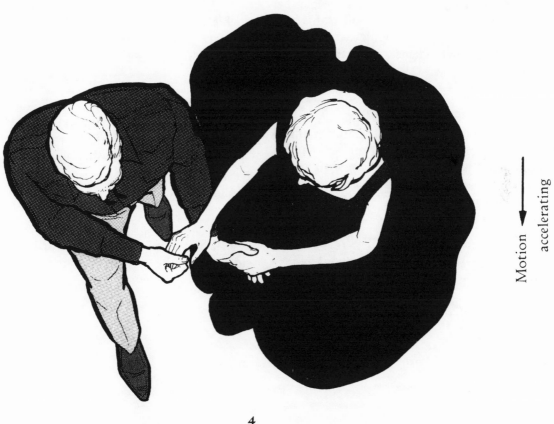

Motion
accelerating

4

Figure 43.   Backtrack (Frames 4 and 5 in a sequence of 5)

# Escort Stance

*Not same as for Promenade*

This is not the same as the stance used for Couple Promenade. It is a different one that presently is used in only one figure—the Wagon Wheel (which is not a fundamental, therefore is not included in this book).

*Same as general-courtesy arm*

The gent and his partner stand side by side and face in the same direction, the gent on the left. He extends his right elbow toward the lady in much the same manner that a gentleman ordinarily offers his arm to a lady for support while escorting her along the street (hence the name of the stance).

*Position of arm*

He brings his right forearm, parallel with the floor, in front of him so that his right hand is in line with the middle of his body. The palm is inclined about 45° to vertical, toward him.

*Lady's left in crook of elbow*

His partner rests her left hand in the crook of his right elbow. Her palm is down,

and the fingers, with the thumb beside them, lightly grasp the upper surface of his elbow joint or the forearm just below it.

*Close but not too close*

The two stand reasonably close to each other, but not so near that the lady is forced to bend her left wrist uncomfortably much to grasp the gent's arm properly.

*Gent presses lady's left*

The gent pulls his right elbow in next to his body enough to press the fingers of his partner's left hand firmly but not painfully against his side.

*What to do with free hands*

He allows his left arm to hang loose at his side. The lady either allows her right arm to hang loose or uses her right hand to hold and work her skirt.

*Use normal step*

The couple move forward side by side, using the normal squaredance shuffle step.

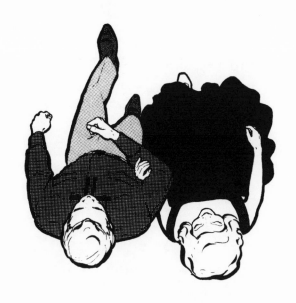

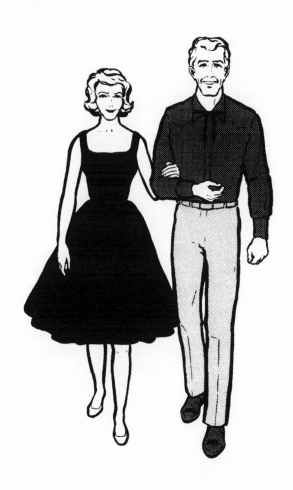

Figure 44.   Escort Stance

# Group 14.   ARCH AND UNDER

## Arch

## Single (Ordinary) Arch

*Side by side*

This maneuver is performed by members of a couple standing side by side and facing in the same direction. They join nearest hands and raise them high enough for other couples or individual dancers to duck down and pass under the Arch formed by the arms.

*Move apart*

As they raise their joined hands to form the Single Arch, they move apart in a short sidestep each, so as to be at two-arms' distance from each other.

*Turn slightly*

In doing so, each customarily turns about ⅛ turn (45°) toward the other. That is, the gent turns 45° to his right, and the lady 45° to her left.

*Makes it easy to watch*

This small shift in direction of facing makes it unnecessary for them to turn their heads excessively while observing the progress of the diving dancers as those dancers pass under the Arch.

*Usually California twirl*

The arching couple almost always initially face out of the set. As soon as the diving dancers have ducked under their Arch, the arching couple—without even lowering their arms—go directly into a California Twirl (described further along in the book). Thus they turn around to face into the set and be ready for the next call.

*Rare exception*

In very rare instances, couples facing into the set will arch. They arch, in the manner described above, long enough for the others to dive thru. But then they do not perform a California Twirl. They simply lower their hands while resuming their parallel facing and normal spacing.

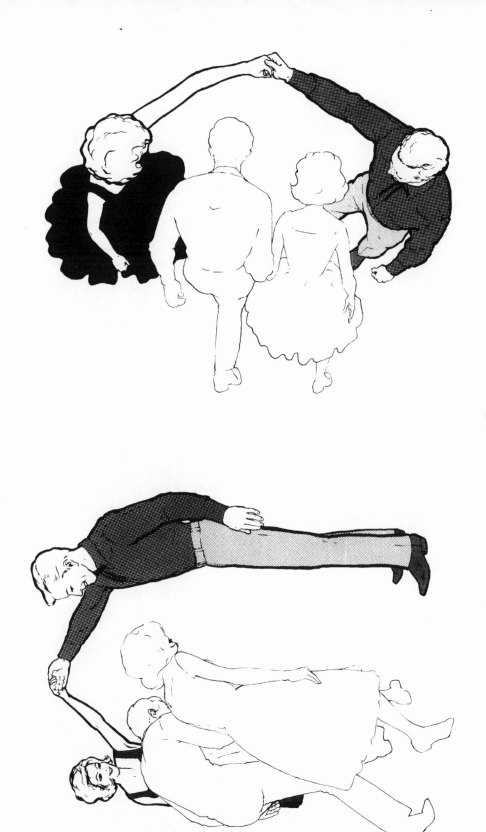

Figure 45. Single Arch

81

# Double Arch

*Members facing*

If the members of a couple are facing, instead of standing side by side, they can form a Double Arch. The gent takes the lady's left and right hands in his right and left, respectively.

*Turn slightly*

As in forming a Single Arch, each partner turns approximately ⅛ turn (45°) so as to make it easier to observe the progress of the diving dancers. But in this situation, since they start out facing each other, the gent turns to his left and the lady to her right.

*Move apart*

Each partner takes a short backstep so that the two of them will be far enough apart, when they lift their joined hands, for other couples (or individual dancers) to have room to duck under.

*Barely grasp, still hardly room*

To make enough room, the partners have to be at a full two-arms' distance from each other, the "grasp" of hands little more than a mere touching of fingers. And even then, unless both partners have exceptionally long arms, there usually is barely enough room for a diving couple.

*Less comfortable than single*

Hence one can see that the Double Arch is a considerably less comfortable-feeling Arch to form than is the Single. And doubtless that accounts for its relative rarity.

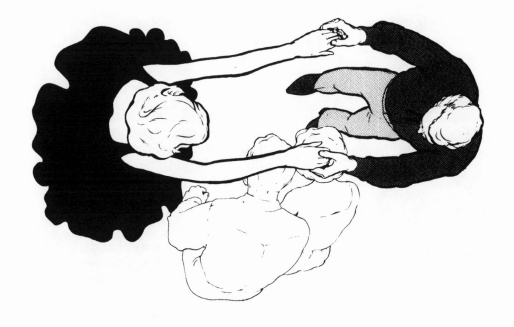

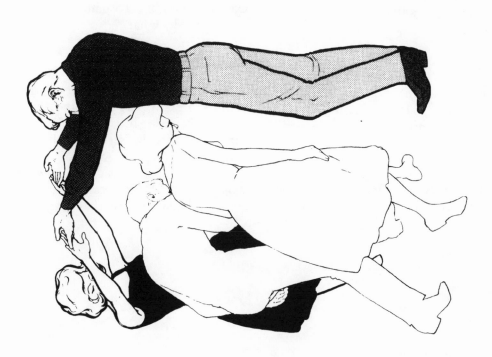

Figure 46. Double Arch

83

# Dive Thru

*Under an Arch*

This maneuver consists in the act of ducking under an Arch, performed by either a couple or a lone dancer.

*Keep holding if were*

If members of a couple are holding hands as they approach the Arch, they continue doing so as they go thru.

*Important general rule*

IT IS VERY IMPORTANT TO REMEMBER THIS GENERAL RULE: In the execution of any maneuver in which some couples arch and others dive under, *almost always the* OUTSIDE COUPLES (THE ONES GOING INTO THE SET) *are the ones who* DUCK UNDER.

*Common occurrence*

In the heat of the moment, while executing a fast figure, the following is quite a common occurrence among beginners.

*Mistake described*

Inside couples, who should be arching, become confused. They try to dive (toward the outside) under an imagined, non-existent Arch of the outside couple, who themselves are ducking (properly) under the missing Arch that the inside couple should be forming but are not.

*Can be bad*

It is easy to see that at best this error occasions some very sheepish expressions on the faces of the inside couple. At worst it can result in some nasty bumps on the heads of both couples.

*Thoughtful callers help*

Prudent callers usually issue supplementary directions, as the figure is being executed, designed to remind the dancers of who is to do what.

*Very rare situation*

In very rare instances the inside couples are supposed to dive thru. When this is the case, it is especially important that the caller be scrupulously careful to give explicit instructions to all concerned to make certain they all know precisely what to do. Helper calls (see Glossary) are doubly helpful in these rare situations.

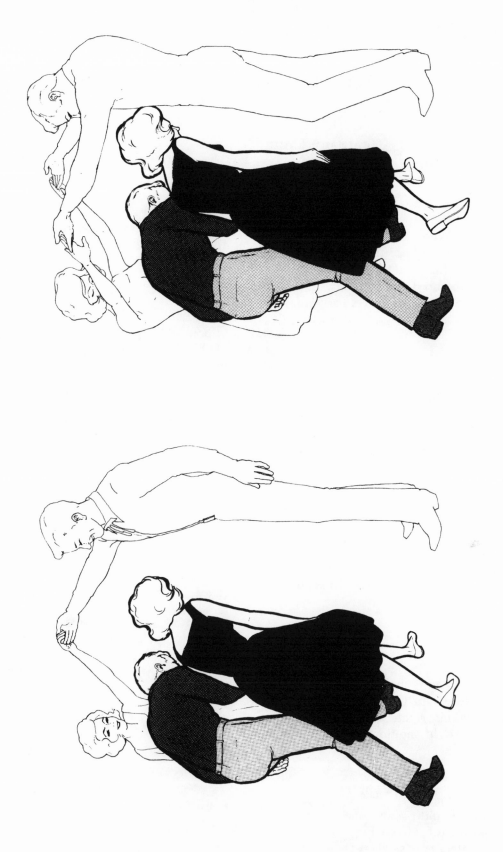

b. *Under Double Arch*

a. *Under Single Arch*

Figure 47. Dive Thru

85

# Group 15. BACK-TO-BACK ENCIRCLEMENTS

## ORDINARY ENCIRCLEMENTS

*Face same way thruout*

These maneuvers are performed by two facing dancers. Thruout their execution, each dancer faces in the direction he faced when he began the maneuver, even though during part of it he moves forward, during part moves sideways, and during part backs up.

*Counts allotted*

One needs eight counts to perform either the Do-Sa-Do or the Seesaw with a person who initially is across the set from him, six counts with a person initially adjacent to him.

*What to do with hands*

The lady may hold her skirt in her hands. The gent may place his hands in the small of his back (although this makes execution of the maneuver somewhat more difficult). Or each may simply allow his arms to hang free at his sides. Occasionally a gent will cross his arms over his chest.

# Do-Sa-Do

*Good to start on left foot*

It is not absolutely essential to do so, but it is very helpful for the dancer to begin this maneuver with his left foot.

*Move to left, pass on right*

As the two dancers move toward each other, each moves slightly to his left, so as to give way on his right, and they pass right shoulder to right shoulder.

*Sideways to right*

After meeting and passing one step beyond, each moves off (from his left foot, of necessity) laterally (sideways) to the right, the pair passing back to back during the lateral motion. Hence the name of this class of encirclements.

*Begin moving backward*

As soon as he has cleared the other person laterally, each dancer begins to move backward, continuing to face in the same direction he faces thruout the entire maneuver.

*Pass left shoulders moving backward*

The pair pass left shoulder to left shoulder as they move backward.

*Veer to left moving back*

As he moves back, each veers to his left enough to bring himself back to his original position, facing the other person.

86

*Reason for starting with left*

Here is why it is desirable to start this maneuver with the left foot. By the end of the second step, the dancer is passing the other dancer right shoulder to right shoulder. By the time he takes his third step, he is beyond the other person and is ready to begin moving sideways to his right.

*On proper foot when needed*

To make an abrupt change of direction to the right, one must move off from his left foot. Thus the advantage of starting on the left foot can be seen: Doing so puts the dancer on his left foot when he has to be on it to do properly what he needs to do.

*Will work, but not so well*

One can start with the right foot and successfully execute a Do-Sa-Do, but he is unlikely to do so in as good form as he will if he starts with his left foot.

*One sideways step enough*

As the dancer is moving laterally (sideways) in one direction, the other person is at the same time moving laterally in the opposite direction. Consequently, just one good-sized step to the side by each suffices to displace them laterally enough to clear each other and allow them to begin moving backward.

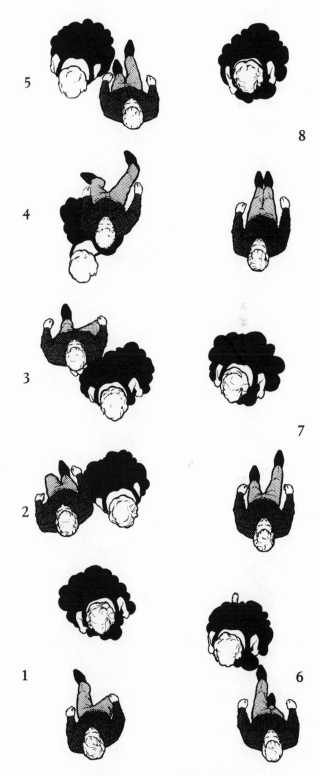

Figure 48. Do-Sa-Do

# Seesaw

*Left-shoulder Do-Sa-Do*

This maneuver is simply a mirror image of the regular Do-Sa-Do. That is, it is a left-shoulder Do-Sa-Do.

*Face same way thruout*

Like the Do-Sa-Do, the Seesaw is performed by two facing dancers, each of whom continues to face in the same direction thruout the performance of the maneuver.

*Good to start on right foot*

It is not absolutely essential that the dancer start with his right foot. But for maximum smoothness and ease of execution, he should lead off with his right.

*Move to right, pass on left*

As the two dancers move toward each other, each moves slightly to his right, so as to give way on his left, and they pass left shoulder to left shoulder.

*Sideways to left*

After meeting and passing one step beyond, each moves off (from his right foot, of necessity) laterally (sideways) to the left, the pair passing back to back during the lateral motion.

*Pass right shoulders moving backward*

As soon as he has cleared the other person laterally, each dancer begins to move backward, continuing to face in the same direction he faces thruout the entire maneuver. The pair pass right shoulder to right shoulder as they move backward.

*Veer to right moving back*

As he moves back, each veers to his right enough to bring himself back to his original position, facing the other person.

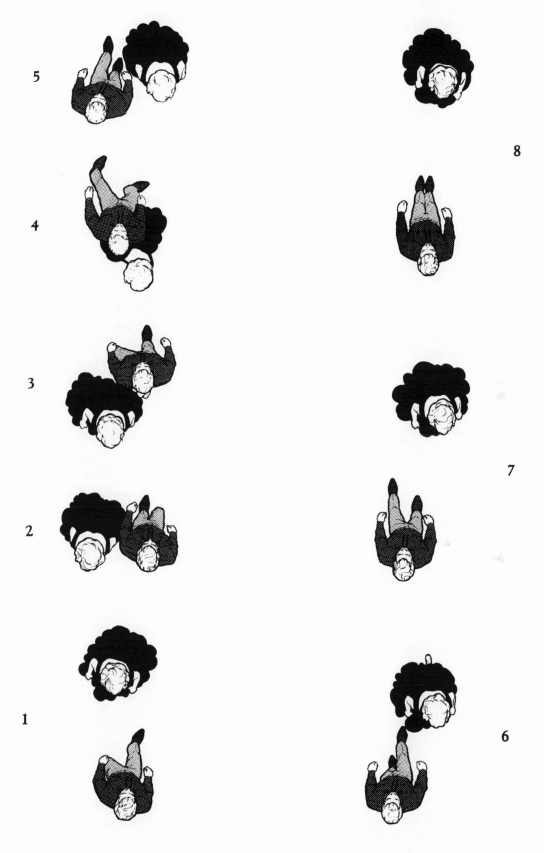

Figure 49.   Seesaw

## 15. Back-to-Back Encirclements

### SPECIAL ENCIRCLEMENTS

*Areas, techniques*

There are several particular ways in which this maneuver can be executed. One is popular in a given area of the country, another elsewhere.

*All basically same*

But they are not radically different. All are similar enough for it to be said, generally speaking, that the maneuver is a variant Do-Sa-Do movement performed with a particular person.

*Often in homes when start*

Often couples are in home positions when the call for this movement is delivered. If they are, the most prevalent procedure is that given here. If they are not, the procedure is altered only as much as necessary, in the circumstances, to enter the maneuver satisfactorily.

*Lady drifts toward center*

The gent turns to face his corner (lefthand lady), but she turns only partway toward him. As he approaches her, she moves forward in the direction she faces. Thus she "drifts" toward the center of the set (toward the gent's right) as they prepare to enter the encircling movement proper.

*Gent can go straight*

Her moving in this direction makes it unnecessary for the gent to move to his left so as to give way on his right as he approaches her, as he ordinarily would.

Because she "gives way for both of them," he can proceed along the same line he started out on (toward her home position) without colliding with her. This makes for a smoother movement.

*Leftface turn moving sideways*

The two do not move across behind each other laterally (sideways) without changing directions of facing, as they do in a normal Do-Sa-Do. Instead, each begins making a leftface turn as he starts moving across laterally behind the other.

*Forward out of encirclement*

By the time each has reached the point where he would begin backing out of a regular Do-Sa-Do, he has already turned ½ leftface turn (180°). Thus he is able to *walk forward* out of the encirclement back toward his home position.

*Customarily seesaw taw next*

The advantage of this technique is that as the dancer comes out of the maneuver and moves back toward home, he already is facing in the proper direction to perform Seesaw Your Pretty Little Taw, which almost always follows next.

*Could back out but doesn't*

One could back out of the encirclement, then spin the proper amount. But that is not the way it is done. It is considerably easier and smoother to do the turning during the crossover, then walk forward out of the maneuver.

# Seesaw Your Pretty Little Taw

*After All Around Lefthand Lady*

This movement almost always is executed immediately after (Walk) All Around Your Lefthand Lady, practically as a continuation of that movement. Nevertheless, it is a separate maneuver, and on rare occasions it is performed by itself.

*Approach from opposite directions*

The gent approaches his home position from the direction of his corner position (the next one clockwise from his home). His partner ("taw") approaches home from the direction of her corner position (the next one counterclockwise from home).

*Lady drifts toward center*

As the two of them near their home position, the lady angles off ("drifts") to her right (the gent's left: toward the center of the set) a slight bit.

*Gent can go straight*

Her doing so makes it unnecessary for the gent to move to his right so as to give way on his left as he approaches her, as he ordinarily would.

Because she "gives way for both of them," he can proceed along the same line he started out on (toward their home po-

sition) without colliding with her. This makes for a smoother movement.

*Rightface turn moving sideways*

The two do not move across behind each other laterally (sideways) without changing directions of facing, as they do in a normal Seesaw. Instead, each begins making a rightface turn as he starts moving across laterally behind the other.

*Forward out of encirclement*

By the time each has reached the point where he would begin backing out of a regular Seesaw, he has already turned ½ rightface turn (180°).

Thus as the dancers complete the encirclement proper, each is prepared to *walk forward* out of it around the ring—the circular course thought of as superimposed within the basic reference square.

*Allemande Left often follows*

The gent is in the *inside* ring (the inner portion of the circular path), facing *clockwise*, and his partner is in the *outside* ring (the outer portion of the circular path), facing *counterclockwise*. Thus they are properly positioned to enter an Allemande Left. Accordingly, it is the maneuver that usually (but not always) follows.

# Group 16.  SASHAYS

At the present time, sashay maneuvers have been almost completely abandoned. Half Sashay and Resashay have been replaced by Rollaway and Whirlaway, the maneuvers making up the next functional group in the book.

*One or other*

Depending upon whether partners are holding hands or have their arms around each other's waist, Rollaway or Whirlaway now is used, the active partner *rolling* across in the appropriate direction.

*Reason for decline*

The reason Half Sashay and Resashay have been supplanted by Rollaway and Whirlaway is that the latter are, relatively speaking, more dynamic movements that are considerably smoother. By comparison, the first two not only are static, but the motions involved are somewhat angular and stiff.

*Mostly in one figure*

Even during the period when they were used, Half Sashay and Resashay were employed, in the main, in one particular figure. Because of the factors mentioned, the figure was quite demanding of the dancers, looking and feeling unsatisfactory unless executed in strict phrase with the music.

*Still fundamentals*

However, regardless of the shortcomings of the three sashay movements, and irrespective of the fact that they are dormant at the moment, they still are distinct and unique ways of transposing partners. Therefore they are true fundamentals and are included in this book with the other fundamentals.

*Might be revived*

Moreover, Resashay, (Go) All the Way Round has not been superseded by any other movement, but has simply fallen into disuse. So far, at least, it has no direct equivalent among the smoother, more satisfying maneuvers currently being used. It certainly is not beyond the realm of possibility that the sashays will someday enjoy a revival of popularity.

# Half Sashay

*Face same way thruout*

This movement consists in an exchange of positions by members of a couple standing side by side and facing in the same direction. Both partners face in this same direction thruout the maneuver, but each moves sideways—and also forward and back a bit—while continuing to face in the original direction.

*Lady in front, gent behind*

The lady moves across to the left in front of her partner, who moves across to the right behind her.

*Counts allotted*

Two counts are needed to complete the Half Sashay.

*Imaginary base line*

For ease in description, we will consider here that a base line exists. It is an imaginary line drawn thru the tips of the toes of the partners as they stand beside each other before commencing the maneuver.

*Right back and to the right*

The gent brings his right foot back from the base line and to the right, diagonally, a distance equal to a fairly large shuffle step. He stops the right foot with the toes slightly farther away from the base line than the heel of the left foot is.

*Left back and to right, then forward*

Next he moves his left foot to the right. Without putting it down, he brings it first back (to clear his partner's feet), then forward until the toes are on the base line. He puts it down six or eight inches to the left of a line thru the heel and toes of the right foot.

*Right straight forward*

Then he moves his right foot straight forward and stops it with the toes on the base line. He now is standing, his feet separated by a comfortable distance of six or eight inches, in the position his partner just vacated.

*Lady opposite*

While the gent is moving as described, his partner does the following. She moves her left foot forward and to the left, diagonally, a distance equal to a fairly large shuffle step. She stops it with the heel a few inches forward of the base line.

Next she moves her right foot to the left. Without putting it down, she brings it first forward (to clear her partner's feet), then back until the toes are on the base line. She puts it down six or eight inches to the right of a line thru the heel and toes of the left foot.

*Gent now on right*

Then she brings her left foot straight back until its toes are on the base line. She now is in the position the gent just vacated. The two of them are in the unusual arrangement in which the gent is on the right and the lady on the left.

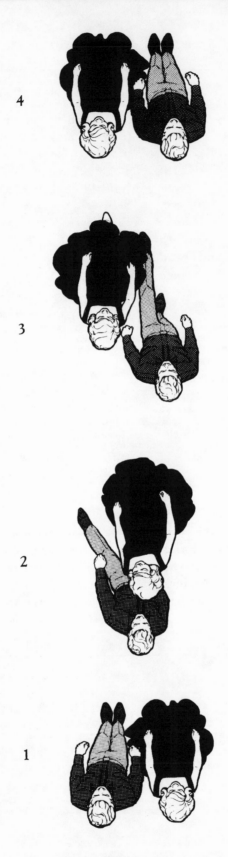

Figure 50.  Half  Sashay

# Resashay

The Resashay is a Half Sashay performed in reverse order, and it always follows a regular Half Sashay. That maneuver places the gent on the right of the lady, standing beside her and facing in the same direction.

*Starts with gent on right*

The Resashay starts from that arrangement and brings the partners back to the original positions they occupied before the Half Sashay was executed—the normal arrangement in which the gent is on the left and his partner on the right.

*Lady again in front, gent behind*

As in the Half Sashay, the lady moves across in front, the gent moves across behind her, and both face in the same direction thruout the maneuver while moving in several directions.

*Counts allotted*

Two counts are needed to execute the Resashay.

*Imaginary base line*

As in the description of Half Sashay, we will consider here that a base line exists. It is an imaginary line drawn thru the tips of the toes of the partners as they stand beside each other initially.

*Left back and to the left*

The gent brings his left foot back from the base line and to the left, diagonally, a distance equal to a fairly large shuffle step. He stops the left foot with the toes slightly farther away from the base line than the heel of the right foot is.

*Right back and to left, then forward*

Next he moves his right foot to the left. Without putting it down, he brings it first back (to clear his partner's feet), then forward until the toes are on the base line. He puts it down six or eight inches to the right of a line thru the heel and toes of the left foot.

*Left straight forward*

Then he moves his left foot straight forward and stops it with the toes on the base line. He now is standing, his feet separated by a comfortable distance of six or eight inches, in the position his partner just vacated.

*Lady opposite*

While her partner is moving as described, the lady does the following. She moves her right foot forward and to the right, diagonally, a distance equal to a fairly large shuffle step. She stops it with the heel a few inches forward of the base line.

Next she moves her left foot to the right. Without putting it down, she brings it first forward (to clear her partner's feet), then back until the toes are on the base line. She puts it down six or eight inches to the left of a line thru the heel and toes of her right foot.

*Gent again on left*

Then she brings her right foot straight back until its toes are on the base line. She now is in the position the gent just vacated. They are once again in the normal arrangement in which the gent is on the left and the lady on the right.

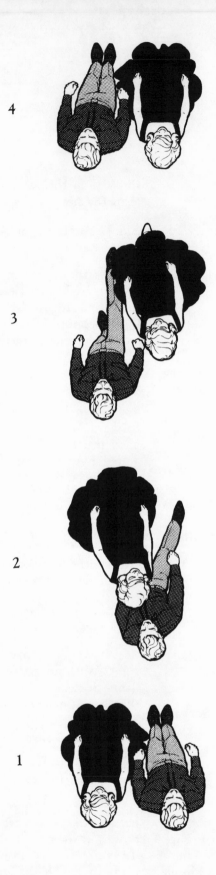

Figure 51.  Resashay

# Resashay, (Go) All the Way Round

Like the regular Resashay, this one always follows a Half Sashay and begins with the gent on the *right* and the lady on the *left*. In the same way, also, both partners continue to face in the same direction thruout the maneuver while moving in several directions.

*Movements in ordinary*

In an ordinary Resashay, partners move clockwise around each other only until they return to the normal arrangement in which the gent is on the left and the lady on the right.

*On around in this one*

This special kind of resashay directs them not only to do that, but also — without stopping — to continue in the same direction (clockwise) till they have moved clear round each other (hence the "All the Way Round") and are back as they began, in the unusual configuration of the gent on the right and his partner on the left.

*Regular plus special*

One might describe this maneuver as a combination of a regular Resashay plus a special resashay in which the gent takes the part of the lady, and vice versa.

*Gent in front in latter part*

In both the Half Sashay and the customary Resashay, the lady moves in front of the gent. But since he takes her part during the latter ("All the Way Round") part of this variant resashay, he moves across *in front of her* during that portion.

*Counts allotted*

Four counts are used in performing this maneuver.

*Imaginary base line*

As in the descriptions of Half Sashay and Resashay, we will consider here that a base line exists. It is an imaginary line drawn thru the tips of the toes of the partners as they stand beside each other initially.

*Left back and to the left*

The gent brings his left foot back from the base line and to the left, diagonally, a distance equal to a fairly large shuffle step. He stops the left foot with the toes slightly farther away from the base line than the heel of the right foot is.

*Right back and to left, then forward*

Next he moves his right foot to the left. Without putting it down, he brings it first back (to clear his partner's feet), then forward until the toes are on the base line. He puts it down six or eight inches to the right of a line thru the heel and toes of his left foot.

*Left straight ahead way forward*

Then he moves his left foot straight forward. However, he does not stop it at the base line beside the right foot, as he would at the conclusion of an ordinary Resashay. Instead he brings it on forward until the heel is a few inches ahead of the base line.

*Right forward, to right, and back*

Next he moves his right foot to the

right. Without putting it down, he brings it first forward (to clear his partner's feet), then back until the toes are on the base line.

*Left to the right and back*

Finally, he brings his left foot to the right and back, diagonally, and puts it down beside the right foot. He now is standing in the righthand position he started from.

*Gent's right shoulder past lady's left*

During his travel, the gent crosses over behind his partner, passes her left shoulder with his right as he moves forward, and then crosses back over, in front of her, into the position he just left.

*Lady opposite*

During that time the lady moves opposite to the gent—to the right and forward, backward, and to the left and forward to the position she just left.

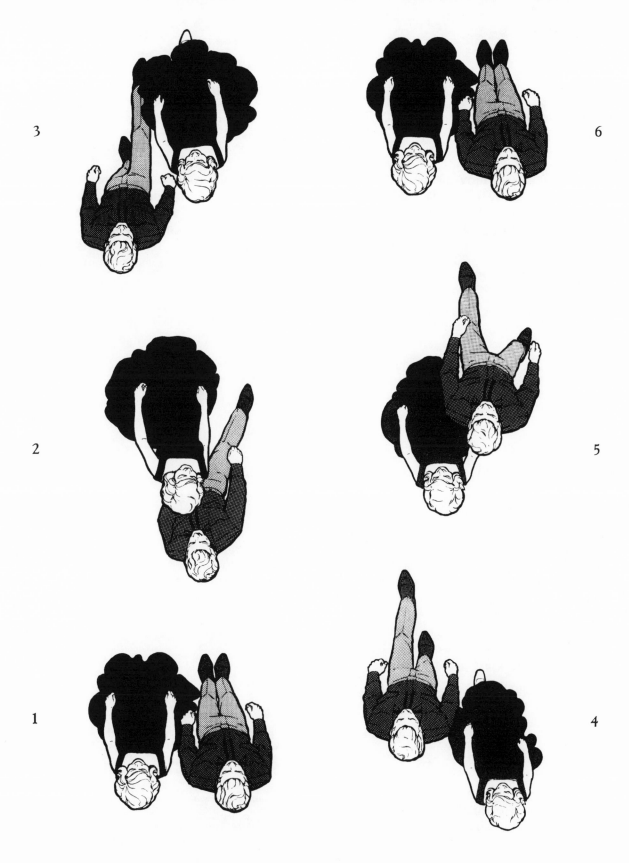

Figure 52. Resashay, (Go) All the Way Round

# Group 17.  ROLL-ACROSS  MOVEMENTS

These two movements (Rollaway and Whirlaway) originally were called Rollaway With a Half Sashay and Whirlaway With a Half Sashay.

*No sidestepping*

The "With a Half Sashay" part of the longer names was somewhat misleading, since no sidestepping of partners, as performed in a Half Sashay, occurs.

*Exchange positions*

"Rollaway" or "Whirlaway" (as appropriate) by itself adequately describes the particular maneuver. The latter part of the original, longer titles merely indicated that in executing either maneuver the dancers exchange positions, as happens in a Half Sashay.

*Counts allotted*

Each of these movements requires two counts to complete it.

# Rollaway

*Fast, smooth exchange*

Rollaway is one of the fastest and smoothest ways for partners to exchange positions while performing certain other maneuvers. They are those, such as Star Promenade and Courtesy Turn (both described further along in the book), in which the partners face in the same direction, side by side, and one of them or both have an arm around the waist of the other.

They usually are moving along, but do not have to be.

*Either may be told to roll*

Rollaway can be performed when the gent is on either side, and either dancer may be called upon to do the rolling. The call is directed to the partner who rolls across. He is the active member of the couple, relatively speaking. He always is a partner whose waist is encircled.

*Gents, ladies, or some of both*

In the Star Promenade this can be either the lady or the gent; in a Courtesy Turn it always is the lady. In an Arky configuration (explained in the article on Star Promenade) it might even be some of both sexes at the same time if, for example, the caller says something like "Outside partners rollaway."

*Inactive member initiates*

The partner who has his arm around the one to whom the call is directed is the inactive member (relatively speaking), but he is the one who *initiates* the action.

*Sideways push, moves closer*

The inactive member gives the active one a slight sideways push in the appropriate direction to start the active member moving across in front of him and around to his other side. At the same time, he begins taking one sidestep directly toward the active member.

*Better for both*

Thus that dancer does not have to travel so far to get onto the path the inactive member was just tracing out. At the same time, the inactive dancer gets onto the other's former path more quickly.

*Full turn*

If the active dancer crosses from right to left, he makes a full (360°) leftface turn as he goes. If he moves from left to right, he makes a full rightface turn.

*Catches with other arm*

As the rolling member passes the halfway point in his travel, the inactive partner anticipates his return on the other side and extends the arm toward which the active member is rolling.

The active partner's movement is such that his back is toward that arm as he moves around to the threequarter point in his passage to the far side of the inactive member.

*Both put arm around*

The inactive member encircles the waist of the rolling partner with his far arm as that dancer, continuing to turn, moves into position on the far side of the inactive partner, slipping his arm around him as he does so.

*Direction initially faced*

The rolling partner ends up on the far side facing in the same direction he initially faced—the direction in which the inactive partner has faced all the while.

*With foot on side headed toward*

For maximum smoothness and ease of execution, the active dancer should start out on the foot on the side he is headed toward.

*Easy to remember and do*

There is nothing at all difficult about either doing this or remembering to do it. The reason is that it is the perfectly natural thing everyone unconsciously does anyway, without even thinking. The foot on the side we are headed toward is the handiest one to start out on, so we use it automatically.

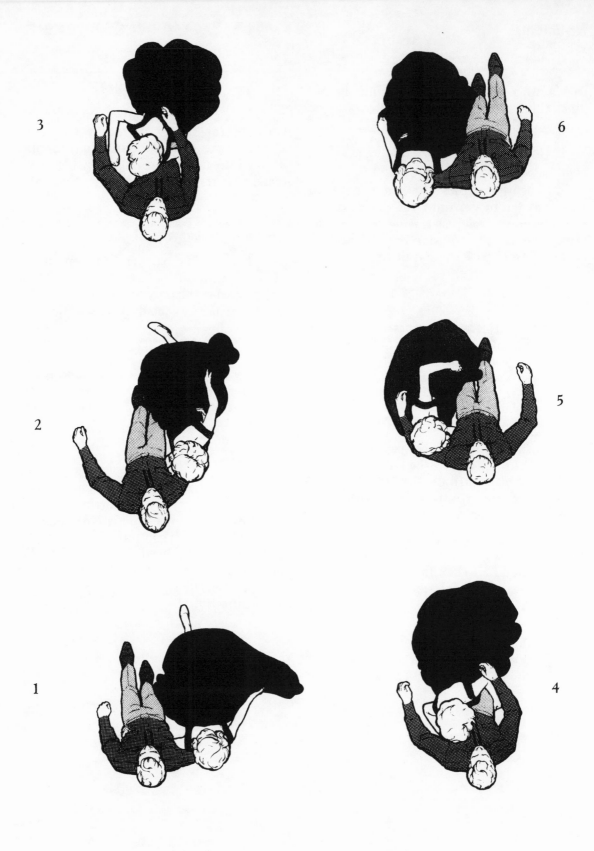

Figure 53. Rollaway (Rolling from Right to Left)

102

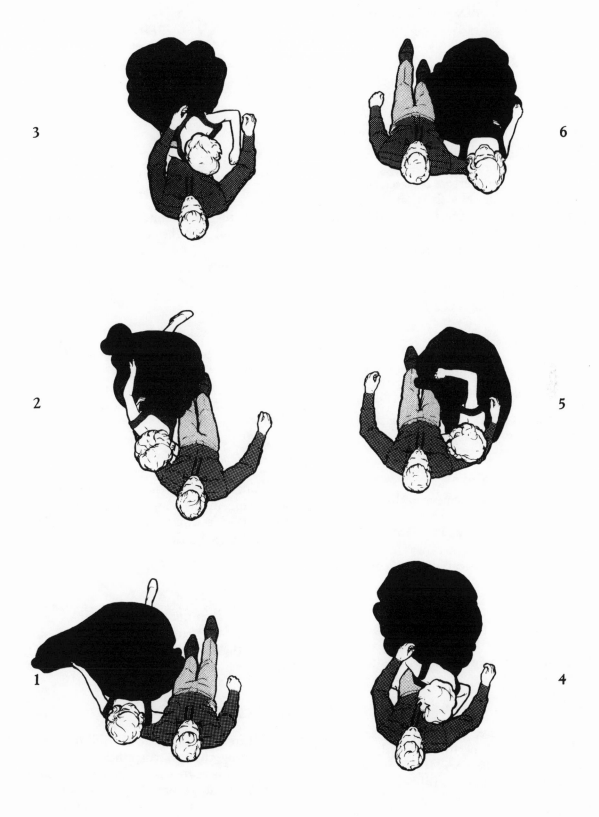

Figure 54.  Rollaway  (Rolling  from  Left  to  Right)

# Whirlaway

*Hands instead of arms*

The only difference between the Whirl-away and Rollaway is that whereas in Rollaway the partners have their arms around each other's waist, in Whirlaway the gent is holding the lady's near hand in his.

The couple are moving along, or sometimes standing, side by side.

*Inactive member initiates*

The partner who rolls across is the active member of the couple, relatively speaking. He is the one the call is directed to. But the action is *initiated* by the *inactive* (relatively speaking) partner.

*Pulls hand across*

The inactive member pulls the active member's near hand across to the left or right, as appropriate, in front of him to start the active partner moving across in front of him and around to the other side.

*Moves toward partner*

At the same time, he begins taking one sidestep directly toward his partner, so that the partner does not have to travel so far.

*Full turn*

If the active member crosses from right to left, he performs a full (360°) leftface turn as he goes. If he moves from left to right, he makes a full rightface turn.

*Both hands momentarily*

As the rolling dancer passes the halfway point in his travel, he will for an in-stant be facing the inactive partner. He extends his free hand, to be taken by the free hand of the inactive member.

At the same time, the dancers retain the original handhold briefly. Thus momentarily each is grasping both of the other's hands.

*Release old, retain new*

An instant later they release the original handhold. But they retain the new hold between what are now near hands as the rolling partner, continuing to turn, moves around to the far side of the inactive member.

*Direction initially faced*

The rolling partner ends up on the far side facing in the same direction he initially faced—the direction in which the inactive partner has faced all the while.

*With foot on side headed toward*

For maximum smoothness and ease of execution, the active dancer should start out on the foot on the side he is headed toward.

*Easy to remember and do*

There is nothing at all difficult about either doing this or remembering to do it. The reason is that it is the perfectly natural thing everyone unconsciously does anyway, without even thinking. The foot on the side we are headed toward is the handiest one to start out on, so we use it automatically.

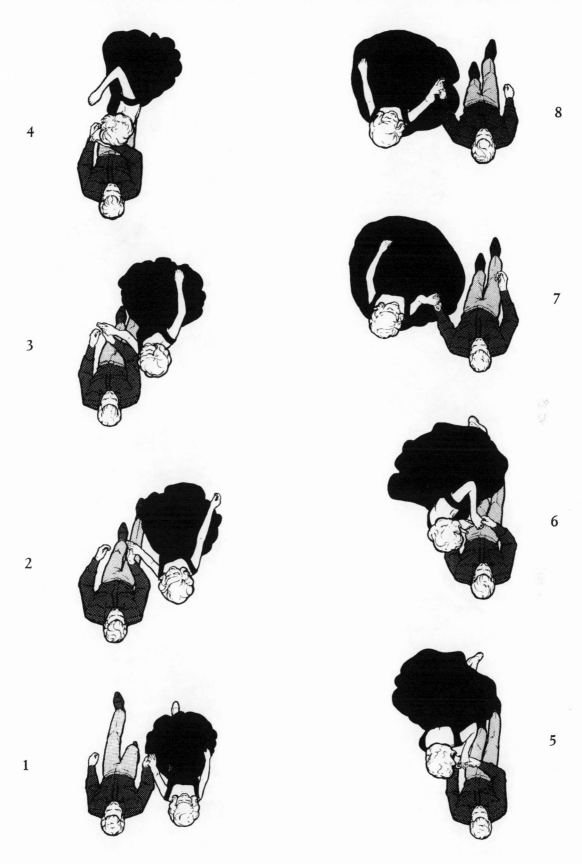

Figure 55.   Whirlaway  (Rolling  from  Right  to  Left)

105

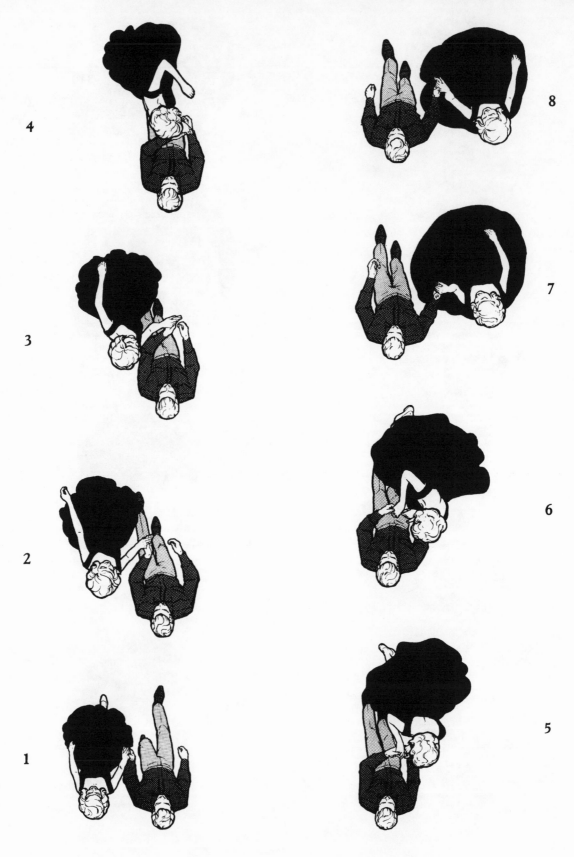

Figure 56.   Whirlaway  (Rolling  from  Left  to  Right)

# Group 18.  STAR THRU

"Loose handhold"

In the execution of maneuvers in functional groups 18, 19, and 20 (Star Thru, California-Twirl Movements, and Box-the-Gnat Movements), joined hands are held high, and the lady turns under them. For convenience in description, it is customary simply to say that "a loose handhold" is employed in those maneuvers.

*Whole series of holds*

That convention is followed in this book, but only because a written description of the hand mechanics would be impracticably long and complicated. For the supposedly simple "loose handhold" actually is a whole series of continuously varying holds. That is, the handhold changes every instant.

*Details impractical*

The dancer soon learns to perform these operations without even thinking about them. Nevertheless, the action in each case is quite complex, and it is not feasible to put very much helpful information into a small number of words.

*Ball and socket*

It can be said only that in general the action is like that of a fixed ball and moving socket, the lady's hand being the ball and the gent's hand the socket moving over and around it.

*Both active, gent's more so*

That is not to say, however, that the lady's hand is static, and only the gent's is active. Both of them move and very definitely are active. However, *relatively* speaking, the gent's hand usually is slightly more dynamic, exerting more of any actual grasping force that may be involved, for instance.

*See pictures*

For a clear understanding of the procedures, the reader is referred to the illustrations of the maneuvers concerned.

# Right (Ordinary) Star Thru

GENT'S RIGHT HAND, LADY'S LEFT

*Pair of dancers*

This is performed by a pair of dancers who face each other. The gent takes the lady's left hand loosely in his right. His left arm and her right are at their respective sides.

*Move to left*

They raise the joined hands and move toward each other, each moving slightly to his left so as to give way on his right.

*Lady ¼ left, gent tight ¼ right*

As she moves forward, the lady turns ¼ turn (90°) to her left, doing part of it under the joined hands. The gent proceeds clockwise around her in a tight ¼ turn to his right, moving behind her back as she turns her body while moving straight ahead.

*Lady moves forward a bit*

As the lady turns, she moves forward a couple of feet in the direction she initially faced. And the gent's movement around her displaces him the same distance forward in the same direction he initially faced.

*In place of other, but side by side*

Thus each ends up in the position the other just vacated. But since each has turned thru ¼ turn (90°), the two are now side by side. Because the lady is on the gent's right, the pair now are partners.

*Establish handhold of Attention*

As the pair are moving into their final positions, they begin bringing their joined hands down. As they are brought down, the gent disengages his momentarily to slip it, palm vertical, under his partner's fingers and grasp them with his thumb in the handhold of Attention. Thus this hold is already established when the hands reach their lowest point.

*Other handhold if appropriate*

Naturally, however, if some other maneuver is to be executed immediately after the Star Thru, the couple do not establish the handhold of Attention, but instead grasp hands in a manner appropriate for the maneuver to be performed.

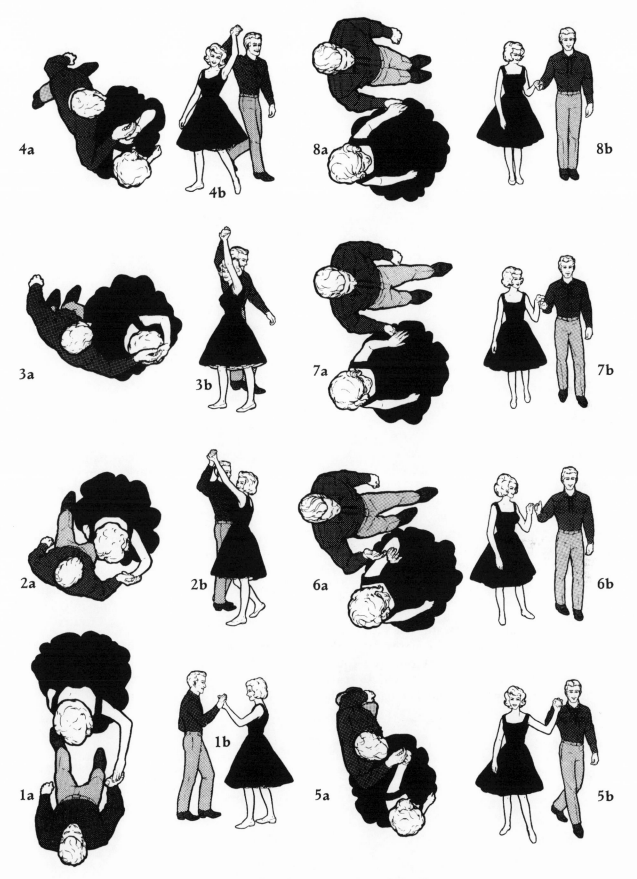

Figure 57. Right (Ordinary) Star Thru

# Left Star Thru

GENT'S LEFT HAND, LADY'S RIGHT

*Less common than regular*

This maneuver is performed by a pair of dancers who face each other, just as the regular (Right) Star Thru is. But it is called far less frequently than that maneuver.

*Reason for rarity*

The reason is that it puts the pair into the unusual arrangement in which the *gent* is on the *right* and the *lady* on the *left*.

*Raise joined hands, move forward*

The gent takes the lady's right hand loosely in his left. His right arm and her left are at their respective sides. They raise the joined hands and move toward each other, each moving slightly to his right so as to give way on his left.

*Lady ¼ right, gent tight ¼ left*

As she moves forward, the lady turns ¼ turn (90°) to her right, part of it under the raised hands. The gent proceeds counterclockwise around her in a tight ¼ turn to his left, moving behind her back as she turns her body while moving straight ahead.

*Lady moves forward a bit*

As the lady turns, she moves forward a couple of feet in the direction she initially faced. And the gent's movement around her displaces him the same distance forward in the direction he initially faced.

*Side by side, gent on right*

Thus each ends up in the position the other just vacated. But since each has turned thru ¼ turn (90°), the pair now are side by side, the *gent* on the *right*.

*Handhold of Attention unless*

As in the regular (Right) Star Thru, the couple establish the handhold of Attention (unless it is inappropriate for the subsequent maneuver) as they are bringing their hands down while moving into their final positions.

But since the gent is on the lady's right, the hold is a mirror image of the normal one and is established with the gent's left hand and the lady's right.

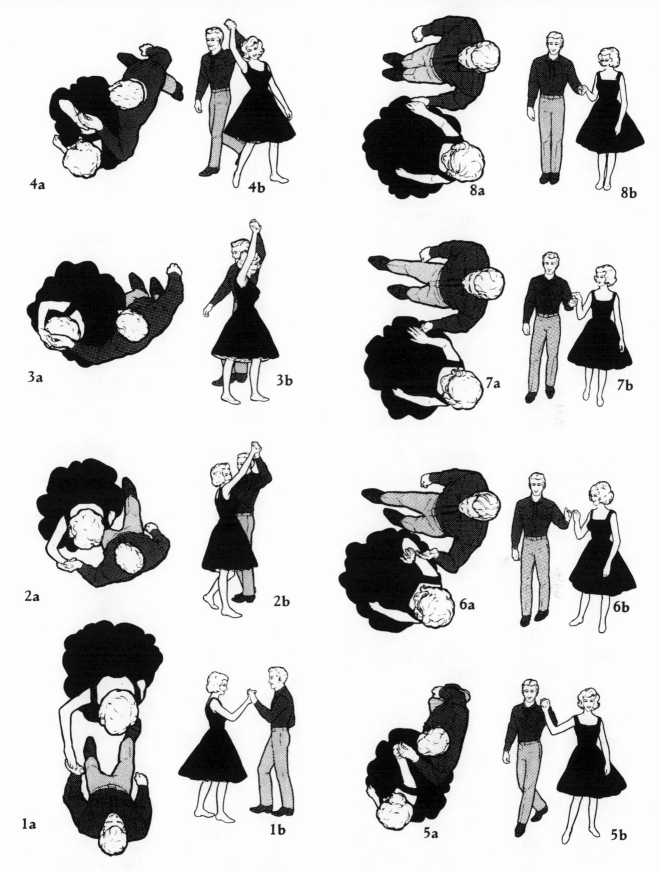

4a 4b 8a 8b

3a 3b 7a 7b

2a 2b 6a 6b

1a 1b 5a 5b

Figure 58.  Left Star Thru

111

# California Twirl

GENT'S RIGHT HAND, LADY'S LEFT

*Like facing, starring thru*

This maneuver also has the name Frontier Whirl. It is a single, separate maneuver and always has been. But in effect it is as if two dancers standing beside each other were to perform two individual movements in rapid succession.

If they should face and immediately star thru, one would have difficulty distinguishing the action from that of a California Twirl.

*Reverse, keeps gent on left*

The California Twirl always begins with a couple standing side by side and facing in the same direction, the gent on the left. It is a fast, smooth way for them to reverse the direction in which they both face, yet keep the gent on the left and the lady on the right.

*Gent very tight half turn right*

The gent takes his partner's left hand loosely in his right. They raise the joined hands, and the gent walks clockwise around the lady in a very tight ½ turn (180°) to his right.

*Lady half turn almost in place*

At the same time, his partner makes a ½ leftface turn, part of it under the raised hands. Although she does not turn in place, she moves only about 18 inches to the left (relative to the way she initially faced) as she turns.

*Exchange positions, direction of facing*

The couple end up facing in the direction opposite that in which they originally faced, but the lady still is on the gent's right. Each is in the position the other just vacated.

*Handhold of Attention unless*

As the dancers are moving into their final positions and bringing their joined hands down, the gent disengages his momentarily to slip it, palm vertical, under his partner's fingers and grasp them with his thumb in the handhold of Attention. Thus that hold is already established when the hands reach their lowest point.

*Other handhold if appropriate*

Naturally, however, if some other maneuver is to be executed immediately after the California Twirl, the couple do not establish the handhold of Attention, but instead grasp hands in a manner appropriate for the maneuver to be performed.

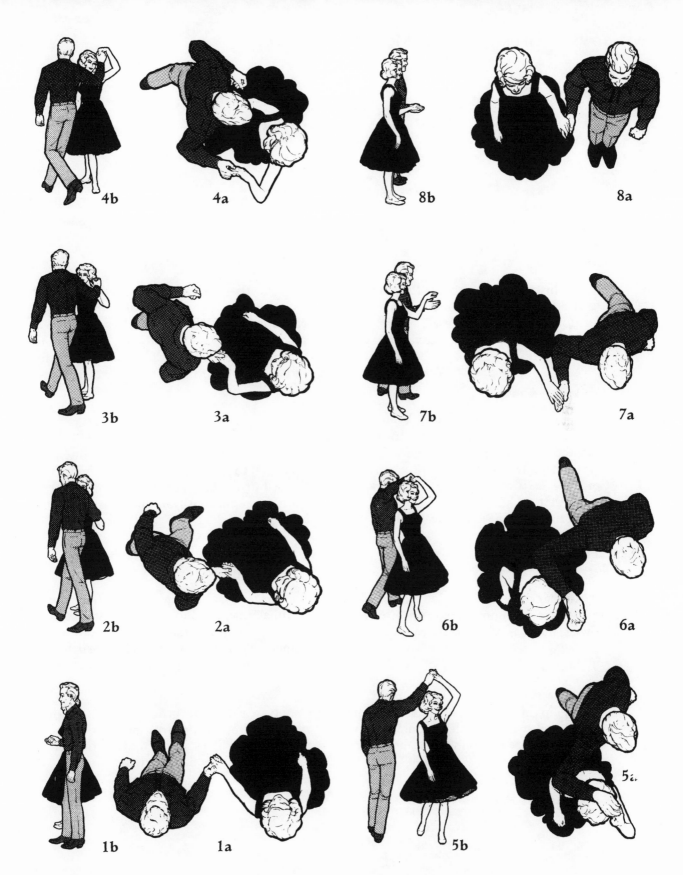

Figure 59. California Twirl

113

# Turn Your Corner Under

GENT'S LEFT HAND, LADY'S RIGHT

*Mirror image of Cal. Twirl*

This maneuver also has the name California Whirl. It is a mirror image of the California Twirl (Frontier Whirl). That is, everything in that maneuver is reversed, right to left.

*Gent must be on right*

Thus the call for Turn Your Corner Under can be delivered only to pairs of dancers who stand side by side, facing in the same direction, the *gent* on the *right* and the *lady* on the *left*. The lady on a gent's left is his corner (lefthand lady); hence the name of the movement.

*Much less common*

Because of the necessary arrangement of the dancers executing it, this maneuver is far less common than the California Twirl, but it is occasionally called.

*Gent very tight half turn left*

The gent takes the lady's right hand loosely in his left. They raise the joined hands, and the gent walks counterclockwise around the lady in a very tight ½ turn (180°) to his left.

*Lady right half turn almost in place*

At the same time, the lady makes a ½ rightface turn, part of it under the raised hands. Although she does not turn in place, she moves only about 18 inches to the right (relative to the way she initially faced) as she turns.

*Exchange positions, direction of facing*

The pair end up facing in the direction opposite to that in which they originally faced, but the lady still is on the gent's *left*. Each is in the position the other just vacated.

*Handhold of Attention unless*

As in California Twirl, the couple establish the handhold of Attention (unless it is inappropriate for the subsequent maneuver) as they are bringing their hands down while moving into their final positions.

But since the gent is on the lady's right, the hold is a mirror image of the normal one and is established with the gent's left hand and the lady's right.

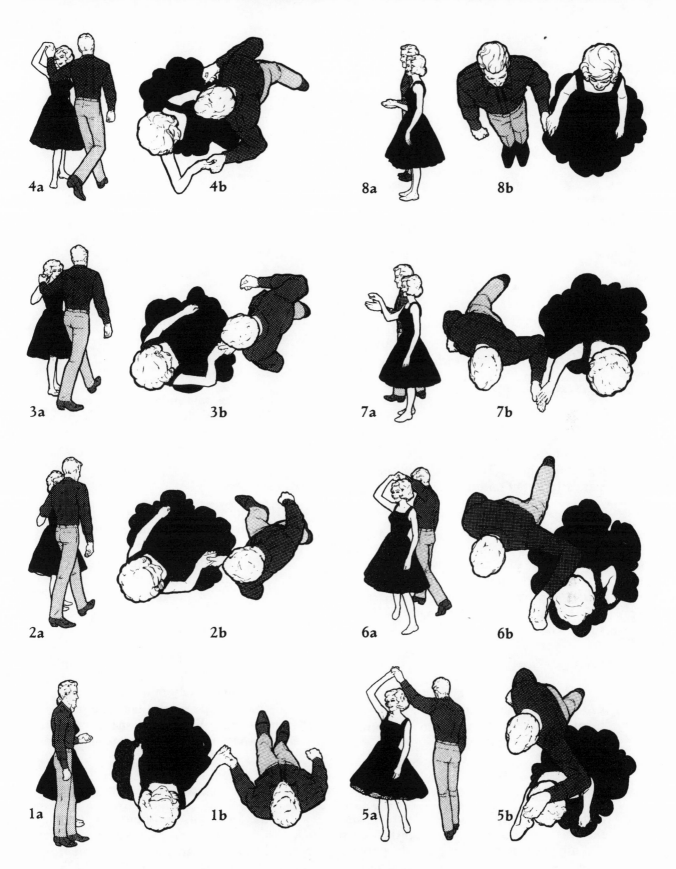

Figure 60.   Turn Your Corner Under

115

# Group 20. BOX-THE-GNAT MOVEMENTS

# Box the Gnat

GENT'S RIGHT HAND, LADY'S RIGHT

*Fast, smooth exchange*

This maneuver is performed by a pair of dancers who face each other. It is a smooth, rapid way for them to exchange positions and directions of facing.

*Joined hands to shoulder level*

The gent takes the lady's right hand loosely in his right. They raise the joined hands to about shoulder level on the gent.

*To left; raise hands higher*

Each moves forward and very slightly to his left so as to give way on his right. As the two approach each other, they raise the joined hands more—high enough for the lady to begin making a ½ leftface turn (180°) as she passes under them.

*Part of lady's turn under hands*

Performing part of the turn under the hands, she continues turning as she moves sideways and backward into the position the gent just vacated.

*Back in, continuing turning*

As the pair draw abreast of each other and the lady begins her ½ leftface turn, the gent begins making a ½ rightface turn. Turning as he goes, he proceeds past the lady, passing behind her back as she turns. He continues turning as he moves sideways

and backward into the position she just vacated.

*Facing again, but exchanged*

Thus the pair end up facing each other again, as they did when they began the maneuver. But now each is in the position the other just vacated.

*Highest as lady starts turning*

The joined hands are at their highest point when the lady begins her turn under them. As the dancers proceed past each other toward their new positions, they gradually lower the hands until they are just above the level of the gent's waist.

*Break, establish conventional*

As can be seen in the illustrations, the grasp is broken at the last instant, and the hands are immediately rejoined in a conventional handclasp much like one uses in shaking hands. What is done next with them depends upon the subsequent maneuver.

*May look strange, but are best*

The series of continuously varying handholds shown may appear somewhat peculiar to the reader. But he will find from experience that they actually are the most practical for this particular maneuver.

116

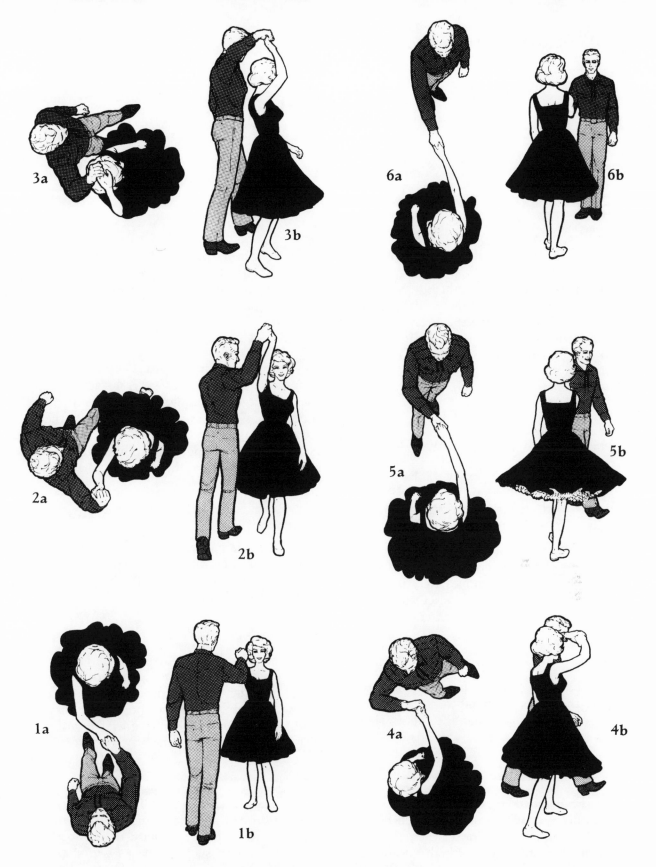

Figure 61. Box the Gnat

117

# Swat (or Box) the Flea

GENT'S LEFT HAND, LADY'S LEFT

*Mirror image, same result*

This maneuver is a mirror image of Box the Gnat. That is, everything in that maneuver is reversed, right to left. However, although the dancers use different hands and turn in different directions in this movement, exactly the same result is achieved: An exchange of positions and directions of facing.

*Uses one or other as needed*

Whenever such a maneuver is needed, a caller uses one or the other of these two as he sees fit—principally as he needs to use the word "gnat" or the word "flea" to rhyme with certain other words in other calls or in his patter (filler material).

If there should be any advantage of one over the other because of the way the dancers are arranged immediately before the maneuver is called, he can select the one that is easier for the dancers to enter.

*Face, raise joined hands*

The pair face each other. The gent takes the lady's left hand loosely in his left. They raise the joined hands to about shoulder level on the gent.

*To right; raise hands higher*

Each moves forward and very slightly to his right so as to give way on his left. As the two approach each other, they raise the joined hands more—high enough for the lady to begin making a ½ rightface turn (180°) as she passes under them.

*Part of lady's turn under hands*

Performing part of the turn under the hands, she continues turning as she moves sideways and backward into the position the gent just vacated.

*Back in, continuing turning*

As the pair draw abreast of each other and the lady begins her ½ rightface turn, the gent begins making a ½ leftface turn. Turning as he goes, he proceeds past the lady, passing behind her back as she turns. He continues turning as he moves sideways and backward into the position she just vacated.

*Facing again, but exchanged*

Thus the pair end up facing each other again, as they did when they began the maneuver. But now each is in the position the other just vacated.

*Highest as lady starts turning*

The joined hands are at their highest point when the lady begins her turn under them. As the dancers proceed past each other toward their new positions, they gradually lower the hands until they are just above the level of the gent's waist.

*Break, establish conventional*

As can be seen in the illustrations, the grasp is broken at the last instant, and the hands are immediately rejoined in a conventional handclasp such as one uses in shaking hands. What is done next with them depends upon the subsequent maneuver.

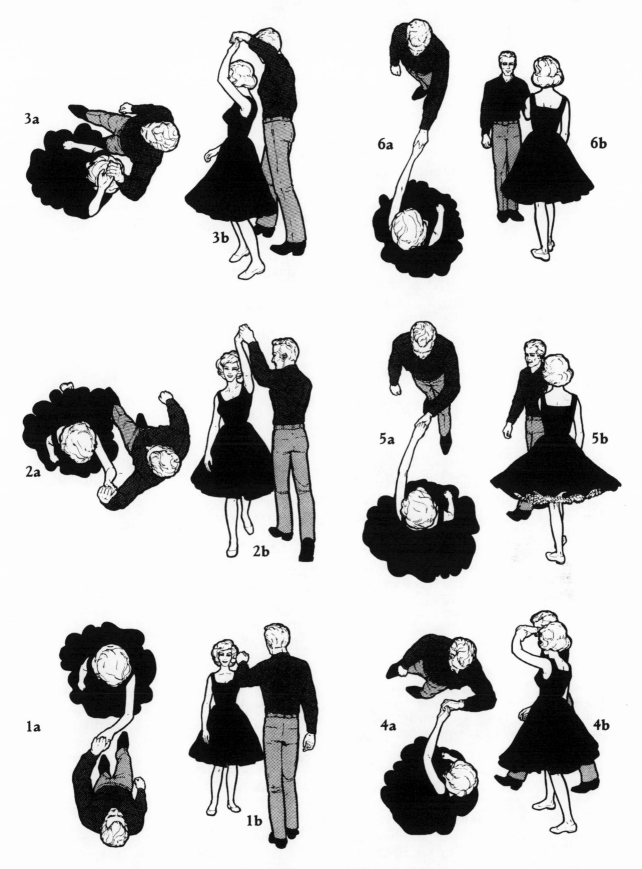

Figure 62. Swat (or Box) the Flea

# Group 21.  COURTESY TURN

*Actually package*

What is called a Courtesy Turn and commonly considered to be a single unit really is a combination, or "package," maneuver consisting of two parts.

*Turn proper unvarying*

It is the second of these that is the Courtesy Turn Proper—the segment in which the gent actually turns the lady. Practically speaking, this part does not vary.

*Three forms of first part*

But the first portion of the combination—the preparatory or entry stage—can have any of three distant forms. That is to say, there are three different ways in which a pair of dancers can *enter* the Courtesy Turn Proper. Each is explained individually below.

*Counts allotted*

All forms of the package require four counts to complete.

## Right-and-Left-Thru Entry

*Couple moving parallel*

In the figure named Right and Left Thru (described further along in the book), the gent and his partner move along parallel with each other, the gent on the left. Anytime the couple are moving in this manner (not just in the Right and Left Thru figure itself), they can enter a Courtesy Turn as follows.

*Left forearm toward lady*

The gent extends his left forearm across in front of him horizontally. His left hand, palm up and slightly toward the lady, is 14-18 inches in front of either his right hip or the right half of his body, at waist level.

*Lady's hands*

The lady puts her left hand, palm down, on the gent's left hand. She can do either of two things with her right hand. She can hold her skirt out with it. Or she can place the back of the hand against the small of her back, next to her right hip.

*Turn proper is Wheelaround*

The couple step ahead with the right foot and then the left. The gent uses his left hand to lead the lady into the Courtesy Turn Proper, which actually is a Wheelaround, rather than an ordinary turn, to the left.

*Minor differences from normal one*

The couple do not have their hands joined in the stance for Couple Promenade, as they do in a regular Wheelaround. And they are slightly closer together, since the gent's right arm is around his partner's waist. Nevertheless, the movement is a Wheelaround, practically speaking.

*Gent uses right hand*

As the gent leads the lady into the wheeling turn with his left hand, he also makes use of his right hand. He pushes gently with it against her right hand (or the small of her back, depending upon what she is doing with her right hand) to make certain of her progress in the turn.

*Headed in opposite direction*

Having completed the sharp, wheeling turn, the couple are headed in the opposite direction from the one in which they last walked in a straight line.

*Possibilities of handholds, movements*

The gent now removes his right hand from his partner's right hand or the small of her back, as the case may be. He may hold one, both, or neither of her hands in one or both of his, depending upon the needs of the maneuver that follows. Likewise, the couple may halt or may continue walking.

*Determines amount of turning*

The exact amount of turning performed in any Courtesy Turn is determined by the demands of the two maneuvers between which it must be fitted—the one that precedes it and the one that follows it.

*Half turn most common*

When the Courtesy Turn is entered in the right-and-left-thru manner, far most often a ½ turn (180°) is performed, as in the description above. The Right and Left Thru figure itself always calls for a ½ turn.

*May be other amount*

But the couple must turn ¾ turn (270°) to end certain figures, and perhaps a different amount to enter others. If there is room for doubt or misunderstanding, the caller usually will specify in some way the amount of turning he expects.

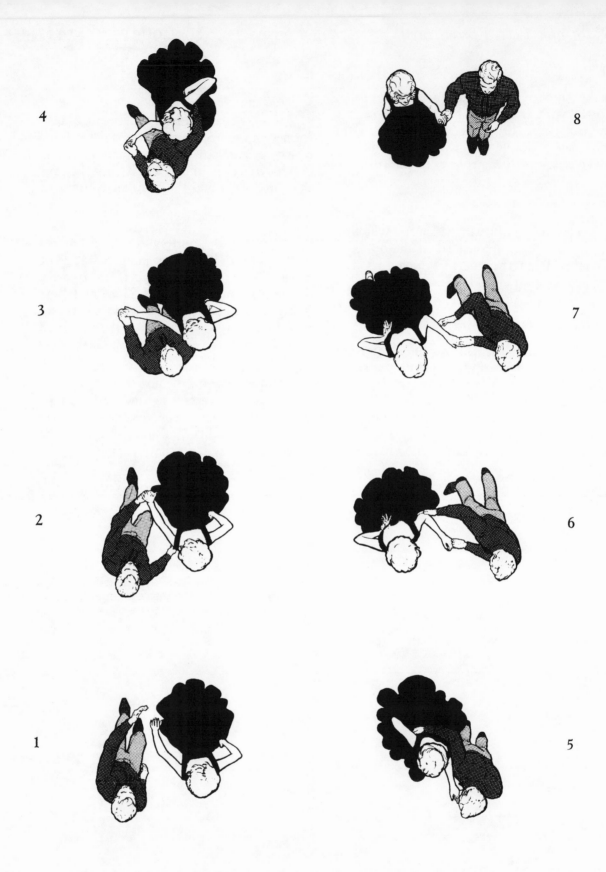

4

8

3

7

2

6

1

5

Figure 63.  COURTESY TURN, Right-and-Left-Thru Entry

122

*Two-Ladies-Chain Entry*

*Stationary, lady approaches*

In the figure named Two Ladies Chain (described further along in the book), the gent is stationary, and the lady advances toward him head on. Anytime this is the situation (not just in the Two Ladies Chain figure itself), a pair of dancers can enter a Courtesy Turn as follows.

*Gent's actions similar*

In general, the gent's actions are quite similar to those of his in the Courtesy Turn begun with the right-and-left-thru entry. But to satisfactorily enter the Courtesy Turn Proper (the part of the maneuver in which he turns the lady), he must alter his technique somewhat.

*Forward, pivots to left*

He anticipates the lady's approach. As she draws near, he should move forward a short step and pivot ⅛-¼ turn (45°-90°) to his left.

*Has to turn only little more*

Thus when she comes abreast of him he has to make only another ¼-⅜ left-face pivot to be by her side and facing in the same direction as she as they enter the Courtesy Turn Proper.

*Usually half turn*

In the Courtesy Turn that is part of the Two Ladies Chain figure, the pair always turn thru ½ turn (180°). Doing so reverses the lady's direction of motion and facing so the gent can send her on back to where she came from if the caller gives the supplementary call "Chain 'em on back."

*May be other amount*

However, the pair may enter a Courtesy Turn in the two-ladies-chain *manner*, but as part of some figure other than the Two Ladies Chain figure itself. If so, they may turn more or less than ½ turn.

*Determines amount of turning*

For the exact amount of turning performed in any Courtesy Turn is determined by the demands of the two maneuvers between which it must be fitted—the ones preceding and following it.

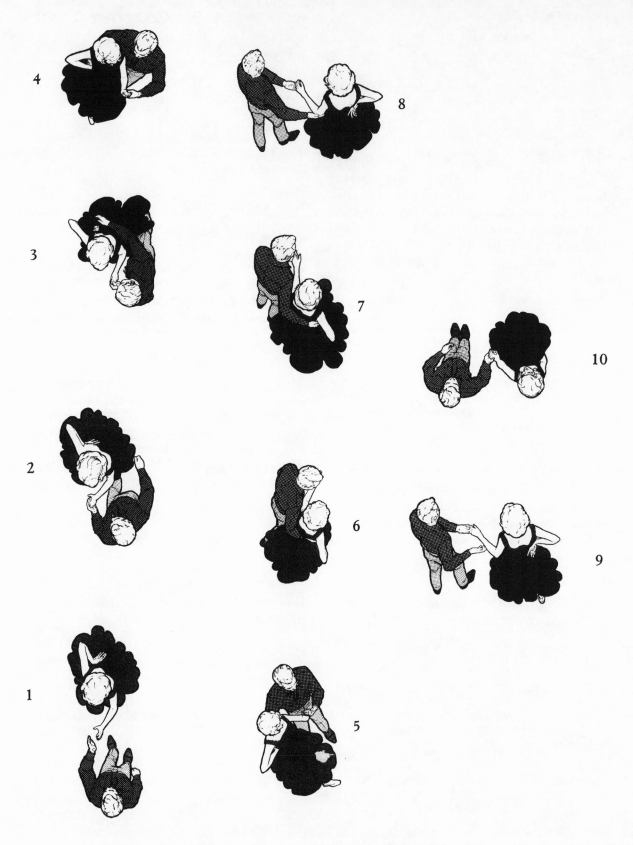

Figure 64. COURTESY TURN, Two-Ladies-Chain Entry

124

## Do-Paso Entry

*Both approaching head on*

The figure named Do Paso is not a fundamental; therefore it is not included in this book. However, in that figure both the gent and the lady move toward each other, approaching head on. Anytime a pair of dancers are moving in this manner (not just in the Do Paso figure itself), they can enter a Courtesy Turn as follows.

*Forearm swing with elbow grip*

The pair establish an elbow grip (a forearm grip will not do) for a Left Forearm Swing. They turn only a very small amount (about $\frac{1}{16}$ turn) in the Swing.

*Gent also turns upper body*

While they are turning in the Swing, the gent, in addition, turns his upper body $\frac{1}{4}$ turn (90°) to the left in respect to the joined forearms.

*Equivalent to anticipatory turn*

He does this so that he can extend his right arm behind the lady's back and put his right hand on her right hand in the small of her back.

This $\frac{1}{4}$ turn is the equivalent of the $\frac{1}{8}$-$\frac{1}{4}$ turn he makes in anticipation, before the lady reaches him, when he begins a Courtesy Turn with a ladies-chain entry.

*Gent $\frac{1}{4}$ turn "behind" as enter*

As the pair enter the Courtesy Turn Proper, their forearms still are joined in the elbow grip for the Forearm Swing, and the gent still is $\frac{1}{4}$ turn "behind" the lady in the way he faces.

*Gent turns lower body extra $\frac{1}{4}$*

He has to face in the same direction as she when they emerge from the Courtesy Turn. To do so, he must—while pivoting thru usually $\frac{1}{2}$ or $\frac{3}{4}$ turn (180° or 270°) in the Courtesy Turn Proper—also turn his lower body (in relation to his head) an additional $\frac{1}{4}$ turn (90°) to the left.

*Sliding grasps down left forearms*

At the same time the gent is doing all the things described above, he must do yet another thing. Relaxing the grasp with his left hand on the lady's left elbow, he changes the hold into a fairly loose, sliding left forearm grip that progresses down her arm toward her left hand. The lady does the same thing with her left hand on his left forearm.

*Moves away as pulls arm out*

In working his grasp down her forearm toward her left hand, the gent pulls her arm out almost straight. To be able to slide the grip down her arm, he moves away from the lady progressively while doing so, increasing the spacing between them a fair amount.

*Open palm under forearm*

As he begins moving his left hand down her left arm, he removes his right hand from her right hand (on her right hip) and places it, palm up, under her left forearm, almost at the elbow. He does not grasp her arm with this hand, but merely slides it along, under her arm, toward her hand.

*Break "grasps" before hands touch*

The gent's left hand never clasps the lady's left. When the sliding grips (his and hers) with the left hands get so low on the forearms that the gent's fingers almost touch the heel of the lady's hand, the pair break the "grasps."

*Handhold of Attention unless*

By this time the gent's right hand, palm up, is under the lady's left wrist. She rotates her hand slightly, so as to be palm down. The gent slides his right hand, palm vertical, under her fingers in the handhold of Attention, unless it is inappropriate for the subsequent maneuver.

*Pair now partners*

Since the lady is on the gent's right, they now are partners—at least for the moment.

*Much for gent to do in four counts*

The foregoing description makes this maneuver sound quite complicated and hard to perform, as far as the gent is concerned. It is. Executing it smoothly and gracefully in only four counts requires considerable skill.

*Most difficult for gent*

However, it can be done; the skill can be developed. With enough practice, any dancer possessed of ordinarily good reflexes can master it.

The beginner can take heart from the knowledge that this is probably the most difficult maneuver he will encounter in squaredancing, and that if he can conquer it, he should be able to cope with any of the others.

*Usually ½, sometimes other*

If the Courtesy Turn begun with a do-paso entry is that which is performed in the *middle* of the Do Paso figure, the pair turn thru ½ turn (180°) in the Courtesy Turn Proper. But if it is the one that sometimes is used to *end* that figure, they turn thru ¾ turn (270°).

*In manner, but not in figure*

Also, the pair may enter the Courtesy Turn in the do-paso *manner*, but as part of some figure other than the Do Paso figure itself.

*What determines amount*

If so, they turn an amount determined by the demands of the two maneuvers between which the Courtesy Turn must be fitted—the ones preceding and following it.

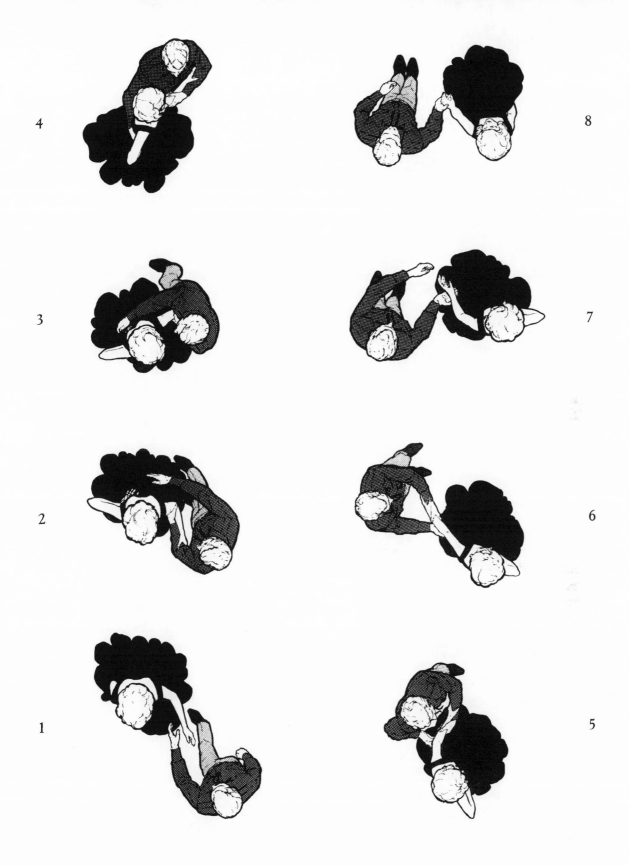

4

8

3

7

2

6

1

5

Figure 65.   COURTESY TURN, Do-Paso Entry

127

# Group 22.  RIGHT-AND-LEFT-THRU  FIGURES

# Right and Left Thru

*Counts allotted*

Six counts are needed to complete the Right and Left Thru if those executing it are already in motion when it is called. Eight are needed if the dancers are stationary when it is called.

*Performed by facing lines*

This figure is performed by facing lines of dancers. Each line consists of either one or two couples.

*May, may not hold hands*

Each gent's partner is on his right. They walk beside each other—usually without touching, but sometimes with the gent holding the lady's left hand in his right. The lines move toward each other.

*Move slightly to left*

As the lines approach, each gent releases his partner's left hand, if he has been holding it, and moves slightly to his left, so as to give way on his right. Each lady also gives way on her right.

*Righthand Pullby*

Each dancer performs a Righthand Pullby with the person he meets. Normally this is a gent with a lady in each case.

*Right-and-left-thru entry*

As soon as the line has progressed beyond the other line, each gent extends his left arm, takes his partner's left hand in his, and courtesy turns her, with a right-and-left-thru entry, into the position just vacated by the corresponding couple in the other line, facing that couple.

*Halt if no more calls*

If no further calls have been given, all couples in both lines halt in place.

*Returns all to initial positions*

But if the supplementary call "Right and left back" is delivered, they perform another Right and Left Thru immediately after the first one, without pausing. This brings all couples back to their original positions.

128

# Two Ladies Chain

*Several ladies-chain figures*

There are at least three ladies-chain figures in squaredancing—Two, Three, and Four Ladies Chain. The last two are not fundamentals, so they do not appear in this book.

*Three Ladies Chain rare*

In addition, Three Ladies Chain is a rather uncommon figure met with only occasionally. Consequently, it almost never is called or referred to except by its full name.

*Shortened titles*

Both Two and Four Ladies Chain are quite common, though. Because of this, oftentimes in casual usage the first word in the title of each is omitted, and the call for either one becomes simply "Ladies chain."

*Seldom really confusing*

This looseness in terminology seldom causes any confusion on the dance floor, because the dancers can determine from their arrangement which figure is more likely to be the correct one.

If they are in facing lines, for instance, it is apparent that *Two* Ladies Chain is the only one that is performable. And if they are standing in home positions it is equally clear that *Four* Ladies Chain is the more feasible of the two figures.

*Good to use full titles*

However, there might be situations in which use of an incomplete title could be ambiguous and lead to confusion. Therefore it is a good idea always to refer to these maneuvers by their full titles.

*Counts allotted*

Two Ladies Chain requires eight counts to execute. The call for it is directed to specified ladies, such as the heads, sides, second and third, or the like.

*Usual positions*

Usually, when the call is delivered, each of the ladies and her partner are either standing beside each other in the stance of Attention or are moving into that position.

*Ushers lady into chain*

Each lady's partner smoothly and gently pushes his right hand (holding her left) away from him and very slightly to the left. Thus he ushers her forward into the Chain.

*Assumes solitary stance*

As soon as she has moved out beyond his reach and disengaged her hand from his, he assumes the stance of Attention for a solitary dancer.

*Very light Pullby*

As they approach each other, each of the two ladies moves slightly to her left, so as to give way on her right. Customarily they perform a Righthand Pullby in which the hands are not grasped, but merely touch. This produces a lighter, daintier appearance than an actual handclasp would

*Other's partner courtesy turns*

Each proceeds past the other to the other's partner, who courtesy turns her ½ turn (180°), so that they face back into the set.

*No pause before "Chain 'em on back"*

If the supplementary call "Chain 'em on back" is given, the lady does not stop or even pause when she faces into the set. Instead, the other lady's partner gives her a gentle push with his right hand (which is still on hers, at her hip), and she goes right back out into the square toward the lady she just chained with.

*Into original position*

They chain once again as described above, and her partner courtesy turns her into her original position, facing into the set.

*Prevalent but poor technique*

Although the following is a very poor technique, all too many gents perform their part of this figure in the way now to be described.

*Gent stays rooted*

When he sends his partner out into the Chain, the gent stays rooted in the position he then occupies. Thus he obliges the lady coming toward him to traverse the entire distance from the other gent by herself. As a consequence, she finds it necessary to take too many steps and too much time in doing so.

*Brief contribution by gent*

But eventually she does reach him. At that time he makes what amounts to practically his sole contribution to the figure in one brief burst of action, courtesy turning her halfway round.

*Makes for uneven figure*

It can easily be seen that when the figure is executed in this fashion it is an un-even, spasmodic one that neither looks good nor feels right to the dancers.

*Should come to meet lady*

The remedy is to smooth it out by having the gent accompany the lady along at least a little more of her path. That is, he meets her partway along her route. He simply steps forward toward her, and to his right, one short step, pivoting about ¼ turn (90°) to his left on his right foot.

*Has to turn only little more*

In doing this, he positions himself such that he has to make only another ¼ or so leftface pivot to be by her side and facing in the same direction she faces. Thus he is able to start moving along with her before she reaches the spot where he turns her.

*Activity spread more evenly*

In this way the activity of the two dancers as a couple is spread out over more of the figure. Consequently, the figure is much less fitful in its execution. Its whole character is altered radically by the gents' taking just one short step forward and to the right.

*Unknown to many*

Oddly enough, however, this simple variation of ordinary procedure is something that many otherwise knowledgeable and competent dancers seem to be totally unaware of.

*Another way to meet and pass*

There is another way for the two chaining ladies to meet and pass by each other. It is less prevalent than the light Pullby, but it deserves to be much more widespread than it presently is, because it is a beautiful way of executing this figure and is a very easy procedure to carry out.

### Two-person Star

The ladies form a palm-to-palm two-person Righthand Star (described in the next functional group) and turn $\frac{1}{4}$ round (90°) in it.

### Turned by other's partner

Immediately after turning 90° to the right in the Star, each lady is turned very nearly $\frac{3}{4}$ round (270°) to the left by the other lady's partner, in the Courtesy Turn.

### Graceful swirling motion

Thus both she and the gent move in a swirling, freeflowing motion extremely pleasing in both its appearance and its feel to those performing it. In addition, the upraised hands are more graceful than the waist-level "grasp" of the light Pullby.

### Gent pivots more

If the two chaining ladies meet and pass in a Star instead of a Pullby, each gent pivots nearly a full $\frac{1}{2}$ turn (180°) to his left, instead of only $\frac{1}{4}$ (90°), as he steps forward and to his right to meet the lady approaching him.

# Group 23.  STAR

The center point of a Star usually coincides with the center point of the set, but not always. For instance, when two or more Stars are executed simultaneously, their centers obviously cannot all be at the center point of the square.

For ease in description, however, a Star at the center is described here.

*What "Star around" means*

The instruction to "Star around" simply means to make up a Star and move around in it the amount specified.

*Lefthand Stars*

Lefthand Stars are just about as common as Righthand Stars, possibly even more so.

# Righthand Star

*Moves in, angles to left*

Two or more dancers designated by the caller step toward the center of the set. If they are moving from home positions, each takes only one or two steps along a direct line between his home and the center of the set. Then he angles to the left so as to begin moving around clockwise the proper distance away from the center point.

*Distance from center*

The proper distance is that which allows him to hold his open hand, palm forward, vertical at the center point of the set and at about face level on a man of average height.

*Arm position*

The upper arm is out to the right almost along a line thru the dancer's shoulders. It is approximately 45° below horizontal. The forearm is a little off vertical.

*Arrangement of hands*

The vertical hands of the dancers are arranged like the leaves of a book opened wide. Preferably they touch at the outer edges of the little fingers.

*Less precise arrangement*

But a less precise arrangement, in which they do not actually touch, but are merely near one another, usually will suffice.

*Palm-to-palm for two*

However, in a Star of only two dancers, the hands always are placed firmly together, the full palms in contact.

*Gent's idle hand*

A gent can either place his idle hand in the small of his back or allow it to hang loose at his side. Holding it in the small of the back feels good to the dancer and gives a smart, sharp look to the starring group. There is no problem because of the elbow's sticking out.

*Lady's idle hand*

A lady often holds and works her skirt with the hand not used in the Star.

Sometimes she lets the idle arm hang loose at her side.

*Walk around spiritedly*

The starring dancers simply walk spiritedly around the center of the Star, clockwise, the fraction of a turn or number of complete turns specified by the caller.

# Back by the Left

*What it means*

The call "Back by the left" tells the dancers in a Righthand Star to reverse their direction of travel and form a Lefthand Star.

*How to do it*

Each dancer has been holding his right hand up to the pivot point. He drops that hand and performs a Turnback, turning toward the *inside* of the set. Lifting his left hand to the center point, he joints in the forming of a Lefthand Star.

*Title misleading*

Note that the wording of the title of this maneuver is misleading. It sounds as if the dancer were being instructed to *turn* to his left to reverse the Star. He is not.

*What call refers to*

The "by the left" refers to the forming of a *Left*hand Star after the dancer has turned around. In turning toward the inside of the formation, he *turns* to his *right*.

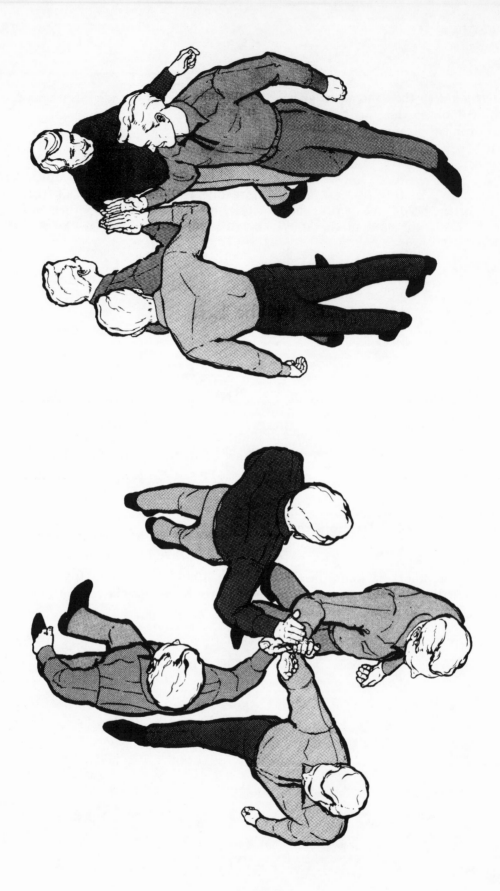

Figure 66.  Righthand Star

# Lefthand Star

*Mirror image*

This formation is a mirror image of the Righthand Star. That is, everything in that maneuver is reversed, right to left.

*Moves in, angles to right*

As the dancer moves in toward the center, he angles to the right to position himself the proper distance from the center point. Holding up his left hand, he moves around counterclockwise.

# Back by the Right

*What it means*

The call "Back by the right," delivered to dancers in a Lefthand Star, means for them to turn to their *left* (the center of the formation) and form a *Right*hand Star.

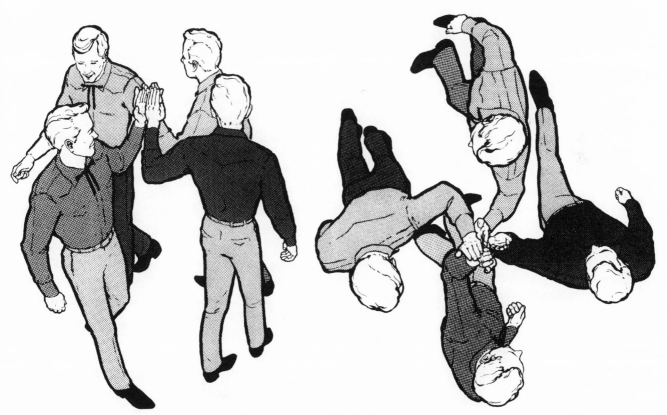

Figure 67. Lefthand Star

# Group 24.  BOX GRIP FOR STAR FORMATIONS

*Don't really join for regular*

Individual dancers acting alone are able to move about very readily. In a regular Star they usually do not actually join their hands at the center, but simply hold them together there, touching along the outer edges.

*Enhances mobility*

The reason is that such an arrangement enhances the dancers' already great mobility, since they can instantly pull their hands away and turn around if a reversal is called.

*Being part of two-person unit awkward*

But when the dancer becomes one part of a two-member unit, his freedom of motion is severely inhibited. In a Star Promenade (described at its own entry, further on), for instance, with his arm around a partner and the partner's arm around him, he discovers that moving in such a fashion is much more awkward than moving alone.

*Especially bad in backup stars*

The same is true, to an even greater degree, when couples have their forearms joined in an elbow grip and one member backs up as the other moves forward beside him, in a backup star (described next in the book). These units are so unwieldy (by comparison) that their members tend to feel downright clumsy while in them.

*Need aid to stability, not mobility*

For this reason, inside partners in such formations discover they do not need a handhold that facilitates mobility. Rather, they find they need one that will give stability to the whole formation by contributing to the steadiness of each couple as they move around.

*Box Grip answers need*

The Box Grip is an extremely firm, rigid hold well suited to the need. Being rigid, it also helps the dancers to maintain the proper spacing between couples as they move around in the rotary formation.

*How to form the grip*

To form the Box Grip, each inside partner extends the appropriate arm (right or left, depending upon whether the formation is a righthand or lefthand one), at about waist level or a little higher, so as to position his hand at the center around which the Star is being formed.

*Arm position*

The upper arm is approximately 45° below horizontal and aligned roughly along a line thru the dancer's shoulders. The elbow is bent, and the forearm, horizontal, is at an appreciable horizontal angle to the upper arm.

*If your arm is the first one*

If the dancer's arm happens to be the first one brought to the center, he waits until the inside member of the couple ahead of him in the formation extends his arm.

Then he grasps that dancer's forearm just above the wrist, fingers on top and thumb on bottom, in a firm but not vise-like grip. The inside member of the couple behind him grasps his lower forearm in the same way.

*Extremely strong grip*

The resulting configuration of hands is strong enough to be used often as a seat in hoisting persons aloft in a sitting position during pep rallies, informal victory parades, and other occasions of elation.

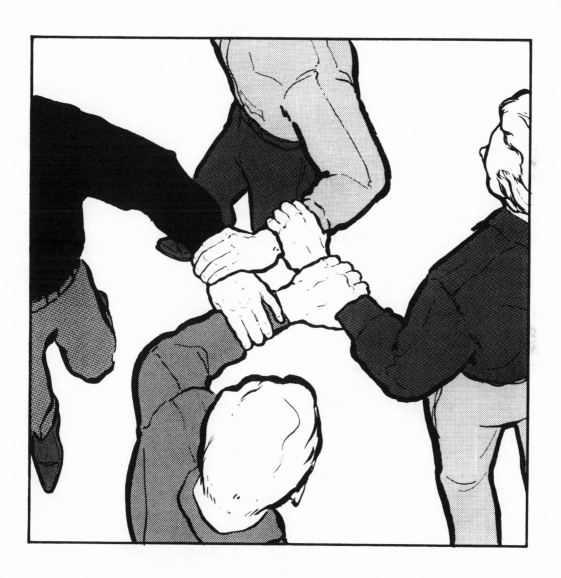

Figure 68.   Box Grip for Star Formations

137

# Allemande Thar

*Forearm Swing with Elbow Grip*

This figure is entered thru a Left Forearm Swing, using an elbow grip. A forearm grip in the Forearm Swing is not likely to prove entirely satisfactory, and a Hand Swing simply will not do.

*Gents usually in center*

Either gents or ladies may be in the center (inside position), as determined by the sequence of calls preceding the Allemande Thar, but gents are more usually there.

*Make Box Grip, back up*

Couples move around in the Left Forearm Swing until the gent is in position to extend his right arm, make up a Box Grip with the other gents, and *back up* in a *right*hand star type of formation that moves *counterclockwise*.

*Retain grasp for Forearm Swing*

The partners maintain the grasp on each other's left elbow joint that they established for the Left Forearm Swing.

*Directions of facing and moving*

The lady remains as she was in the Swing—beside the gent, but facing in the opposite direction. Therefore when he begins backing up counterclockwise on the inside of the formation, she *walks forward* counterclockwise on the outside to remain beside him.

*Discontinuing backup star*

The Allemande Thar (backup) Star is discontinued by executing the maneuver called Shoot the Star (described later in this section).

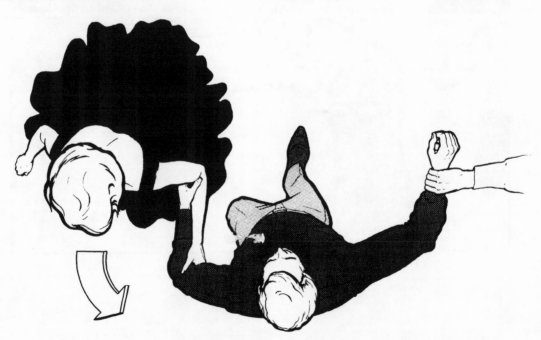

Figure 69. One Couple in an Allemande Thar Backup Star

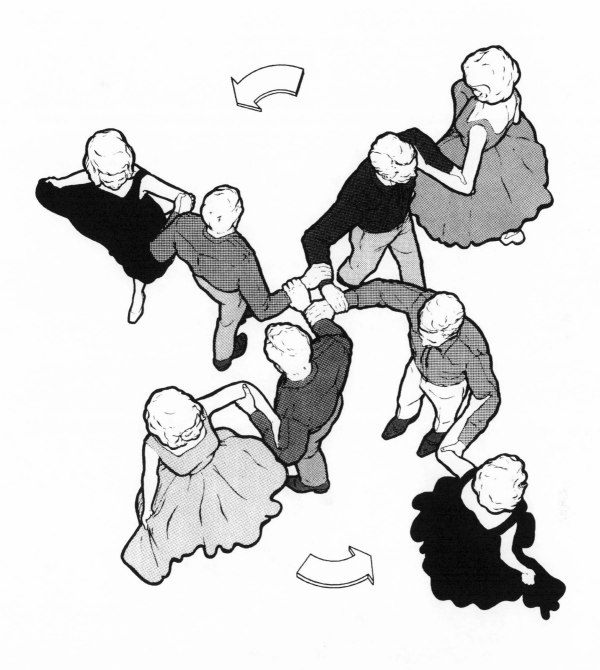

Figure 70. Allemande Thar Backup Star—Entire Formation

# Wrongway Thar

*Mirror image*

This figure is a mirror image of the Allemande Thar. That is, everything in that maneuver is reversed, right to left.

*Directions of facing and moving*

Thus it is a *left*hand star type of formation in which the inside partner backs up *counterclockwise*. Naturally the outside partner must walk forward clockwise to remain beside the partner on the inside.

*Forearm Swing with Elbow Grip*

The Wrongway Thar (backup) Star is entered thru a Right Forearm Swing, using an elbow grip. A forearm grip in the Forearm Swing is not likely to prove completely satisfactory, and a Hand Swing simply will not do.

*Discontinuing backup star*

The Wrongway Thar is discontinued by executing the maneuver called Shoot the Star (described next in this section).

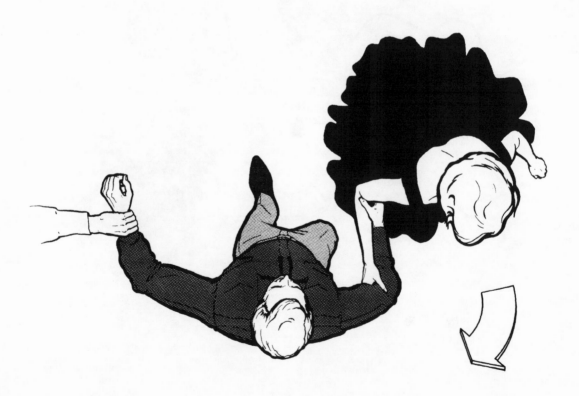

Figure 71. One Couple in a Wrongway Thar Backup Star

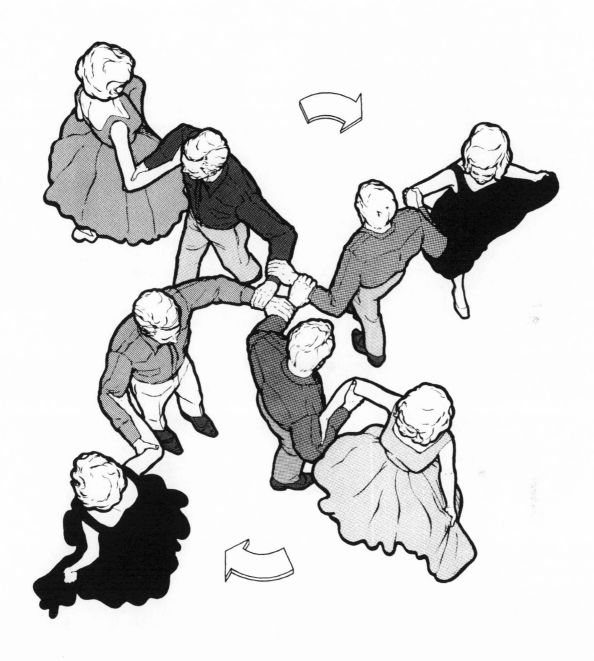

Figure 72. Wrongway Thar Backup Star—Entire Formation

# Shoot the Star

*Discontinues backup star*

The function of this movement is to discontinue a backup star and take the dancers into some other maneuver.

*End Box Grip, do Forearm Swing*

The inside partner (who usually is the gent) disengages his hand from the Box Grip at the center of the star, and the couple perform a Forearm Swing—left out of an Allemande Thar, right from a Wrongway Thar.

*Turn halfway round unless*

Unless otherwise instructed, they turn halfway round (180°). But if the basic call is modified by a supplementary instruction, as in "Shoot that star, with a full turn around," they turn the amount specified.

*Still facing in opposite*

The partners release forearms as they finish turning, but continue to face in opposite directions. When they go into the next maneuver, each moves forward in the direction he faces.

# Throw in the Clutch

*Transforms into two figures*

This maneuver transforms a backup star into a conventional Star surrounded by a Promenade in Single File moving in the opposite direction to it.

*Release forearms; insides stop, go other way*

When the call is given, couples release the forearm hold, and the inside partner halts smoothly, keeping his hand in the Box Grip at the center.

Then, without turning, he immediately begins moving in the opposite direction, reversing the motion of the rotary formation.

*Facing same way, but moving differently*

Since he previously was backing up, he is still facing in the same direction he has been facing all along. But now he is mov-

ing forward, instead of backing up, as he faces in that direction.

*Outside partner does nothing different*

When her arm is released, the outside partner (who usually is the lady) does nothing whatever different from what she has been doing. She does not turn, but simply continues to move forward in the same direction in which she has been moving all along.

Now, though, she is promenading in single file. Thus the partners now are both moving forward, but in opposite directions.

*Promenade in Single File around Star*

Until further instructions are given, the set of inside partners continues rotating as a Star, and the outside partners continue promenading in single file in the opposite direction around the Star.

# Group 26.  STAR PROMENADE

This figure, in the right or the left form, is performed far most often by four couples, but occasionally by three, and sometimes by only two.

*Ways couples can be disposed*

Within each couple, the members can be disposed in any of the following ways.

1. Gent on the left, lady on the right (the normal arrangement).

2. Lady on the left, gent on the right.

3. Gents in both positions, or ladies in both.

*Arky arrangements*

The last two are called *Arky* (for Arkansas) configurations. Arky arrangements in the Left Star Promenade are not common, but they are not remarkably unusual, either.

*Rule instead of exception*

But reversed positions in the Right Star Promenade probably are the rule, rather than the exception, since the ladies seldom are on the inside.

*Left more common than right*

The Left Star Promenade is definitely more common than the Right Star Promenade.

*How to reverse direction*

Dancers engaged in a Star Promenade reverse its direction of rotation by executing the maneuver called Hub Backs Out, Rim Goes In (described later in this section).

# Left Star Promenade

*Arm around waist*

Each member in each couple places an arm around his partner's waist. The couples walk counterclockwise around a center point in a circular pattern, making up a rotary formation.

*Box Grip best*

At the center of the formation, the in-side hands of the inside dancers sometimes are held so as to touch along their outer edges, as in a regular Star.

But the Box Grip (described previously, at its own entry) is much more satisfactory, because of the greater stability it affords the couples.

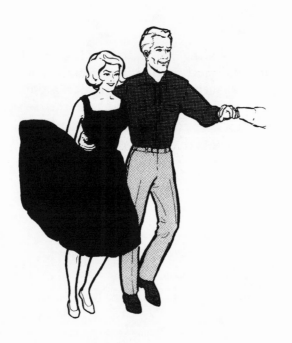 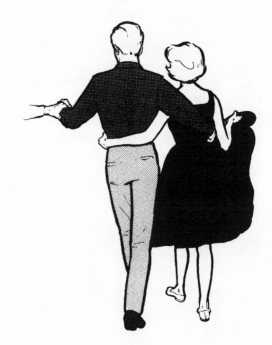

Figure 73.   One Couple in a Left Star Promenade

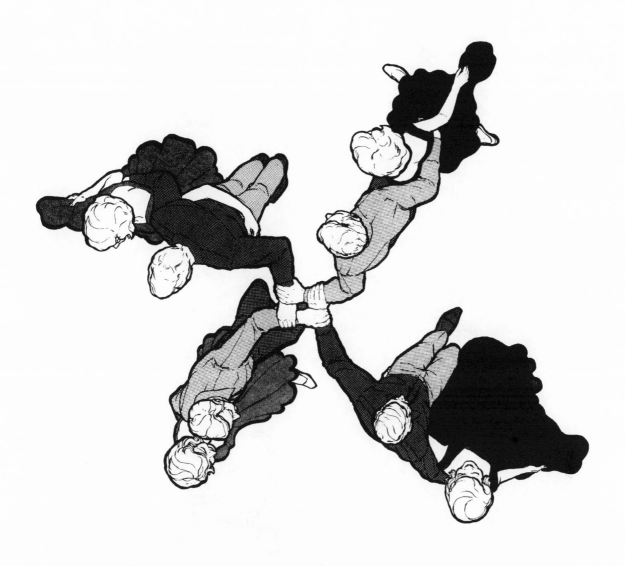

Figure 74.   Left Star Promenade—Entire Formation

145

# Right Star Promenade

*Usually formed by reversing left*

Although this figure is not as common as the Left Star Promenade, it is not notably unusual, either. Most often it is formed by reversing a Left Star Promenade.

*Gents usually inside after reversal*

The reversal is accomplished by executing Hub Backs Out, Rim Goes In (described later in this section).

Usually (but not always) that maneuver is followed by some call such as "Ladies rollaway" to place the gents on the inside of the formation.

*Will be mirror image*

If both those maneuvers are performed, then the Right Star Promenade will be a mirror image of the Left Star Promenade. That is, everything in that latter figure will be reversed, left to right, including the positions of the members within each couple.

*Mirror image most common*

This type of Right Star Promenade, with the gents on the inside of the formation, is considerably more common than the one with the gents on the outside.

*New Box Grip*

Inside members use their right hands to make up a new Box Grip, and the couples move around clockwise.

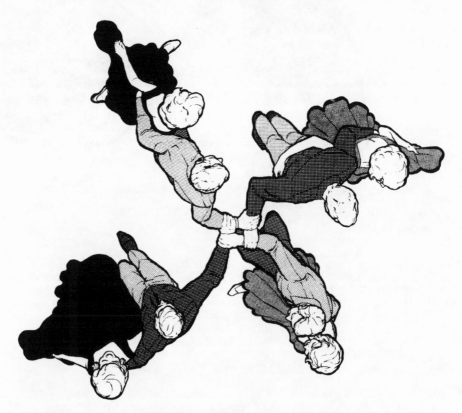

Figure 75.  Right Star Promenade—Entire Formation

# Spread the Star Out Wide

*Not ordinary Star*

The star referred to in the title of this maneuver is not an ordinary Star composed of individual dancers, but a Star Promenade made up of couples.

*Remove arms, join hands*

When the call for the movement is given, the couples continue moving in the same direction, maintaining the star formation. However, the members of each couple remove their arms from around each other's waist and join the hands of those arms.

*Move apart*

Continuing to move beside each other in the rotary formation, the two dancers smoothly move apart until their bodies are almost as widely separated as they can be while hand contact is maintained.

*Still parallel in circular path*

That is, the partners now are at very nearly two-arms' distance from each other, still holding hands. They still are facing along their circular path in the same way and moving parallel with each other. Each arm is bent just enough to be comfortable.

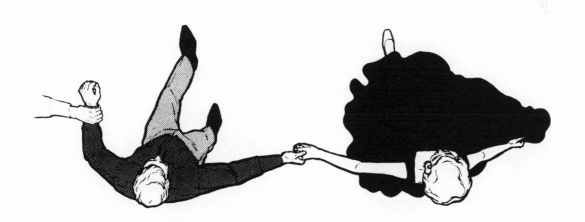

Figure 76.   One Couple in a (Left) Star Promenade Spread Out Wide

# Hub Backs (or Flies) Out, Rim Goes In

*Reverse rotation of star formation*

This movement is also called Gents (or Ladies, as appropriate) Back Out, Ladies (or Gents) Swing In. Its function is to reverse the direction of rotation of a Star Promenade.

*Usually gents in hub, ladies in rim*

Usually the gents are on the inside (in the hub) of a Star Promenade, and the ladies on the outside (in the rim). But the opposite arrangement is not remarkably unusual.

*Break Box Grip, arm still around*

Each of the inside partners releases his hold with the hand in the Box Grip at the center of the formation. But he does not take his other arm from around his partner on the outside.

*Each couple wheels around*

Acting as a unit, each couple executes a movement identical with a regular Wheelaround except for the fact that the dancers are not holding hands, as they are in the Promenade Stance.

*Half turn in some areas*

In some areas it is customary to wheel no more than the ½ turn (180°) of the regular Wheelaround maneuver. But to many dancers, wheeling only ½ turn does not have a satisfying feel to it, because it seems unfinished and incomplete.

*1½ turns more prevalent*

For this reason, it probably is more generally customary for the couple to wheel on around an additional full turn, for a total of 1½ turns. Either ½ or 1½ turns brings them to the position where the dancer who has been on the outside now is on the inside, and vice versa.

*New Box Grip, move forward*

As soon as the wheeling is finished, the partner now on the inside does his part in making up a new Box Grip. At the same time, the couple begin moving forward, causing the star to rotate in the direction opposite that in which it formerly rotated.

*Caller often specifies*

If the caller desires the dancers to wheel thru 1½ turns, and wants to make sure they do not break off after only ½ turn, often he will specify in his call to "Make a full turn around." Here the word "full" is only nominal; it means not just one turn, but 1½.

# Break to a Line

*Gent usually breaks*

This maneuver is executed by a Circle of any number of dancers, but most often three or more. Gents usually break, but on occasion ladies do. The word "Break" in the title actually refers to two different but closely associated things.

*Breaks with left hand*

Ordinarily, the person specified or indicated by the call releases the hand he has been holding in his left hand, but continues to hold the one in his right. Thus he *breaks* (severs) *the Circle* with his left hand. (In special circumstances the dancer breaks with his right hand, but this is very rare.)

*From Circle into straight line*

At the same time, he *breaks out of, or away from, the circular path* to lead those following behind him into a straight line facing into the square. Thus he breaks the Circle itself and (usually at the same time) also breaks *out of* it to a straight line.

*Places it along proper side of square*

The convention is that if head gents break, each does so in such a way as to place his line of dancers along a side of the square containing one of the side home positions (number 2 or number 4).

If side gents break, each places his line along a side of the square containing one of the head positions (number 1 or 3).

*Leaves Circle at right point*

The gent departs from the circular path at a point such that he will be able to properly position his line along the appropriate side of the square. Of course he is aided considerably in this by the caller's delivering the call at the right moment.

*Along side next counterclockwise*

He should proceed along a course such that he can halt near the far end (as he progresses) of the side of the square *next counterclockwise* from that side containing the home position from which he left when the Circle was formed.

*Example*

For example, say heads (with their partners) go out to the right and circle up four, then break to a line of four. The number one gent's line will be along the side of the square containing home position number 2, and the number 3 gent's line will be along the side containing position number 4.

*Positions line symmetrically*

Each gent breaking to a line should take into consideration the number of dancers in the Circle (which becomes a straight line) and choose his stopping position so as to make the line symmetrical about the center (the home position) of the side of the square along which the line is formed. He is at the left end of the line formed, as viewed by its members.

149

*Most back up; some move sideways*

As the members of the Circle becoming a straight line progress toward their final spots in the line, some of them find it necessary to move slightly sideways. During the latter part of the maneuver, most of them have to back up a bit.

*Too much crack the whip*

If a line of more than three were formed in just this way, its length would force the last dancer to move backward very rapidly, because of the crack-the-whip effect.

*Forward until last moment*

To avoid this, she (for it usually is a lady) does not back into position all the way. Instead she moves in a special way that makes it possible for her to walk forward until almost the last moment, then whirl into place.

*Progressive leftface turn*

Her partner is holding her left hand. As they leave the circular path, they gradually lift their joined hands higher than her head. She makes a leftface turn—slowly at first, then faster.

*Arm nearly straight out*

Near the beginning of her turn, her left arm is very nearly straight out in front of her. She keeps it in this position for a moment as she walks toward her spot in the line.

*Moves under own arm*

As she nears the spot, however, she fixes her left hand in space, above the dance floor, and moves under it.

*Bends elbow, swivels wrist*

To do this, she must bend the elbow more and more as she goes under, her hand loosely joined to her partner's right hand and swiveling in wrist action as she begins to turn rapidly.

*Under Arch and backs up*

As she passes under the Arch formed by her arm and her partner's arm and completes a little more than ¼ leftface turn, she backs up a step or two into place beside her partner, on his right. While she is moving into place, they begin lowering the joined hands.

*Break, establish conventional*

As they are doing so, the gent disengages his hand and regrasps hers in a form of the basic handhold of Attention appropriate to an Ordinary Straight Line having the spacing that has developed.

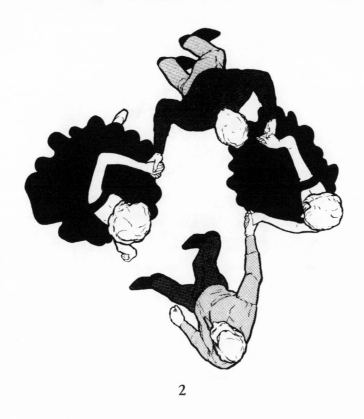

2

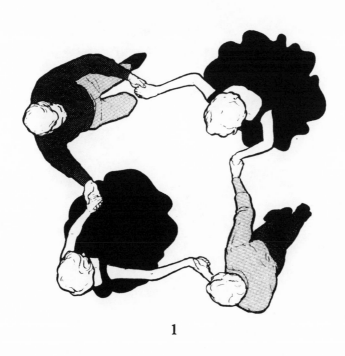

1

Figure 77. Break to a Line (Frames 1 and 2 in a sequence of 8)

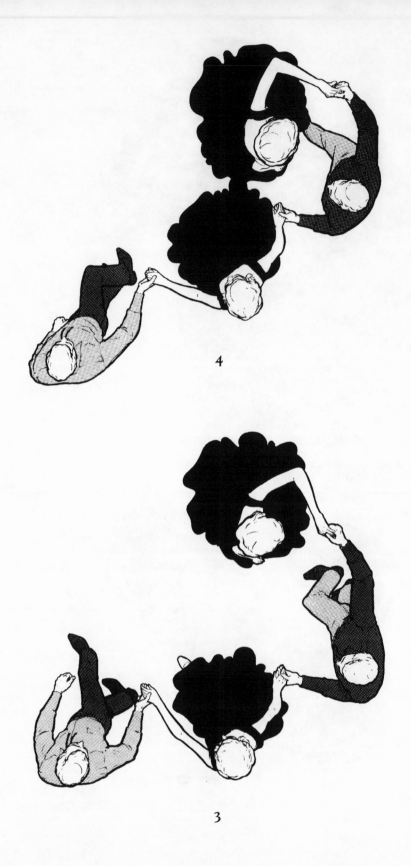

4

3

Figure 78. Break to a Line (Frames 3 and 4 in a sequence of 8)

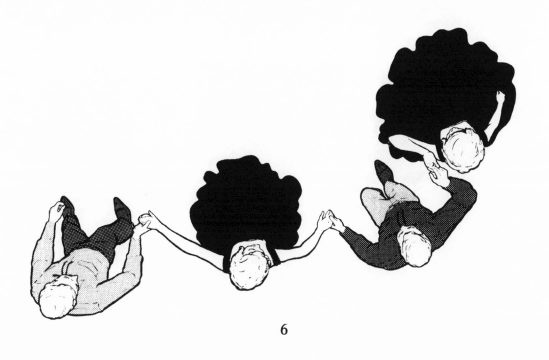

6

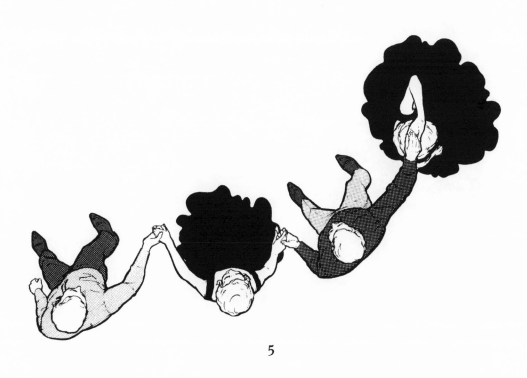

5

Figure 79.   Break to a Line (Frames 5 and 6 in a sequence of 8)

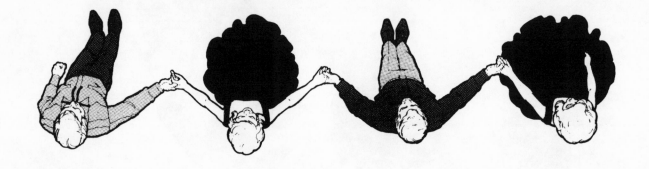

8

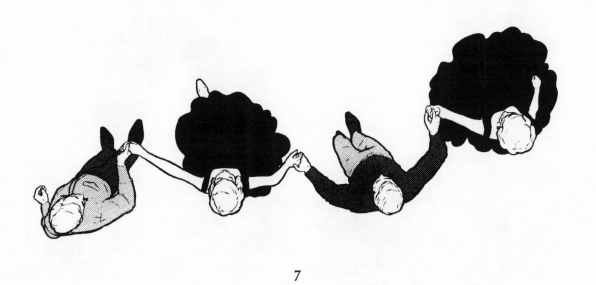

7

Figure 80. Break to a Line (Frames 7 and 8 in a sequence of 8)

154

# Rip and Snort

*Begun from Circle*

This figure is begun from a Circle—usually of all eight dancers—moving in either direction, but far most commonly clockwise. When the call is given, the rotation of the Circle slows smoothly and stops.

*Lead out before stops*

Even before it halts, however, the designated couple, its members moving beside each other, lead out across the Circle, taking the other dancers with them. Everyone continues holding hands.

*Opposite couple arch*

When the leads reach their opposite couple, those dancers raise their joined hands in an Arch so the leads can duck under.

*Leads under, separate*

As soon as the leads have dived under the Arch, they drop hands and separate. This breaks the Circle, which by now is considerably deformed.

*Draw rest thru*

The gent goes to the left, the lady to the right, and the two of them draw the rest of the Circle thru behind them. All, except for the leads, still are holding hands.

*Slightly larger circular path*

In leading his side of the broken, extremely distorted Circle around to the left, the gent moves in a tight turn around his opposite lady and immediately enters a circular path roughly the same as the original one, but just outside it (that is, slightly larger in diameter), moving counterclockwise.

*Partner same but to right*

Similarly, his partner moves in a tight turn to the right around her opposite gent, immediately entering the same circular path just outside the original one, and moving clockwise.

*Next two pairs not partners*

The next two pairs of dancers to pass under the Arch formed by the couple opposite the lead couple are not partners. In the first, the gent is a member of the lead couple's righthand couple, and the lady is from their corner couple.

In the second, the gent is from the corner couple, and the lady is from the righthand couple.

*Just move beside each other*

In each instance the two dancers are not holding hands with each other, but merely moving along beside each other while each holds hands with those ahead of him and behind him in the severely warped Circle.

*Opposite couple begin pivoting*

As the last two dancers other than themselves go thru, the members of the opposite couple, who are arching, must pivot rather rapidly. The gent has to pivot to the right, and the lady to the left, to maintain their handhold (which must be kept loose) and preserve the continuity of the misshapen Circle at that point.

*Pivot becomes pirouette*

After all the other dancers have passed under the Arch made by the opposite couple, the members of that couple must do so themselves, continuing to hold each other's hand. They do this by continuing the pivoting they began when the last pair started to duck under. At this point it actually becomes a pirouette, rather than a regular pivot.

*Pirouettes toward arm in Arch*

As he pirouettes, the gent holds his right arm fixed in the same position in space, above the dance floor. His chest moves closer to it as he turns. His left arm is pulled under his right and around his body to the right by the person holding his left hand.

*Raises arm in Arch*

Eventually he no longer can hold his right arm straight. He then bends it at the elbow and raises it over his head. But he keeps his forearm in a direct line to his partner, maintaining the Arch.

*Under own Arch, lowers arm*

Ducking his head under his right forearm and continuing to pirouette, he turns under his own Arch formed with his partner. As soon as he has completed a full rightface turn (360°) and is facing into the new Circle (still broken, but now undistorted), he drops his right arm to the same level as the left one.

*Partner same in mirror image*

While the gent is turning under the Arch he is helping to form, his partner is doing the same thing in mirror image. She moves her left arm in similar fashion as she pirouettes thru a full leftface turn.

*Meet at home, join hands*

At the completion of the figure, the members of the lead couple approach their home position from opposite directions around the broken but now again undistorted Circle. When they meet there, they join hands to form an unbroken Circle once again.

*Start circling if no call*

The caller will specify the next maneuver to be performed. But in the absence of immediate instructions, the dancers all begin moving clockwise, in an ordinary Circle once more, as soon as the lead couple join hands.

*Sometimes form facing lines*

Occasionally the caller will instruct the dancers to break and form two (facing) lines of four, instead of another Circle, from the Rip and Snort.

*End handhold after pirouette*

In such an event, the members of the pirouetting opposite couple break their handhold with each other after the pirouette, and each half of the Circle (lead by one of the leads) moves out into a line tangent to (touching) the original Circle, its members facing into the set toward the members of the other line.

*"Any old couple rip and snort"*

Sometimes the call "Any old couple rip and snort" is given. This is a stimulating and enjoyable figure, but the dancers must approach it with a degree of caution.

*Must be careful*

A couple leading out in response to the call must do so decisively and without delay. But at the same time they must keep an eye out for possible action by other couples in the set.

Otherwise it might be that one or more of those others are leading out at the same time, each active couple heedless of what the others are doing. If they are not observant, a collision is almost certain to ensue.

*Awareness all that is needed*

Even four-way crashes have been known to happen. These occurred in sets in which exuberant member couples failed to monitor the actions of the other couples as they *all* simultaneously initiated the execution of this delightful but slightly dangerous figure.

All that is needed to assure perfect safety, though, is alertness in observation.

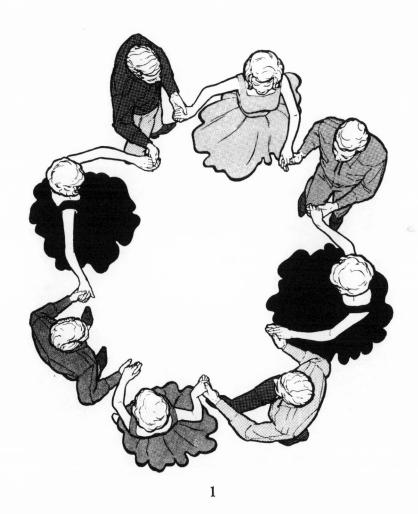

1

Figure 81.   Rip and Snort (Frame 1 in a sequence of 13)

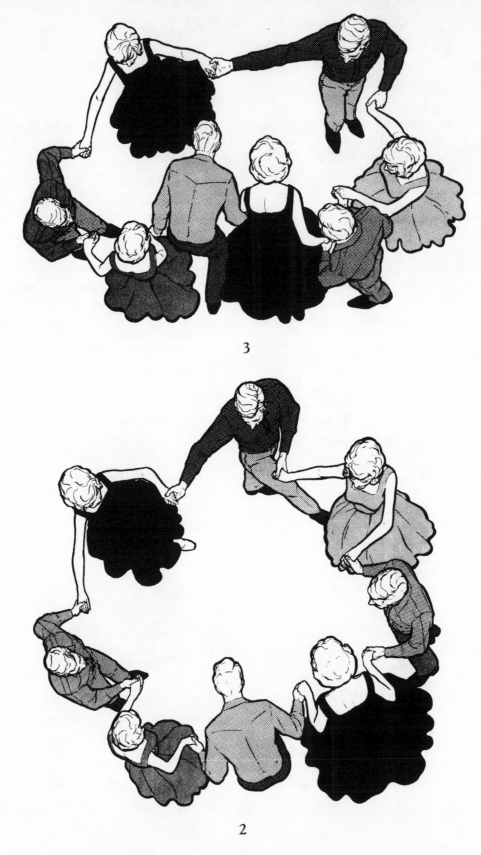

3

2

Figure 82. Rip and Snort (Frames 2 and 3 in a sequence of 13)

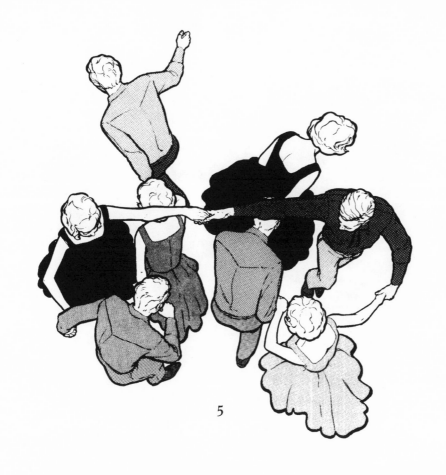

5

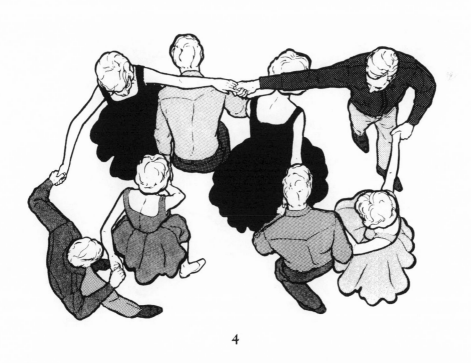

4

Figure 83. Rip and Snort (Frames 4 and 5 in a sequence of 13)

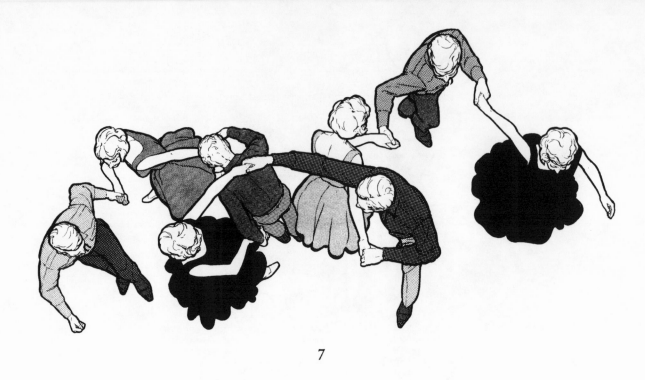

7

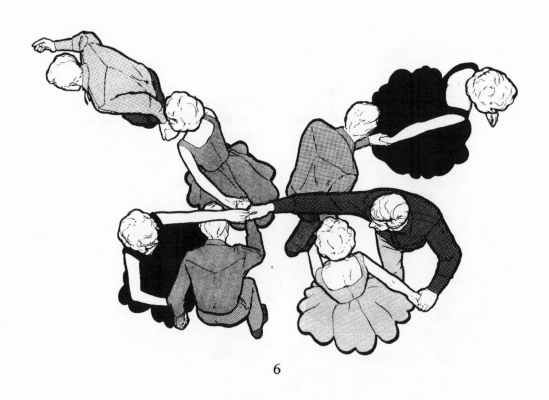

6

Figure 84.   Rip and Snort (Frames 6 and 7 in a sequence of 13)

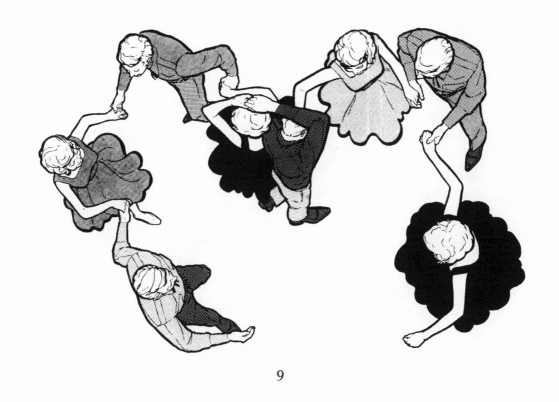

9

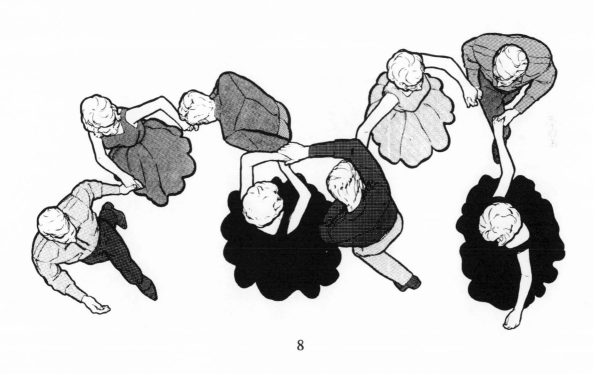

8

Figure 85.  Rip and Snort  (Frames 8 and 9 in a sequence of 13)

161

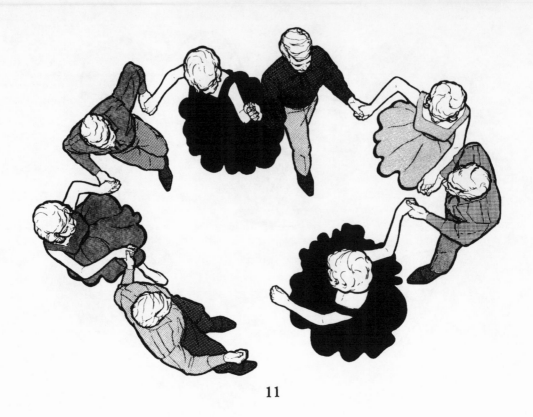

11

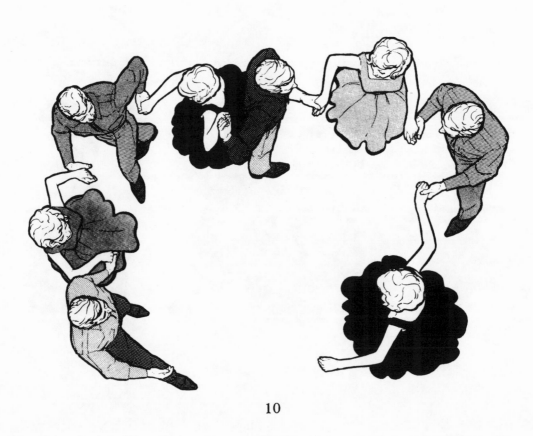

10

Figure 86.  Rip and Snort  (Frames 10 and 11 in a sequence of 13)

162

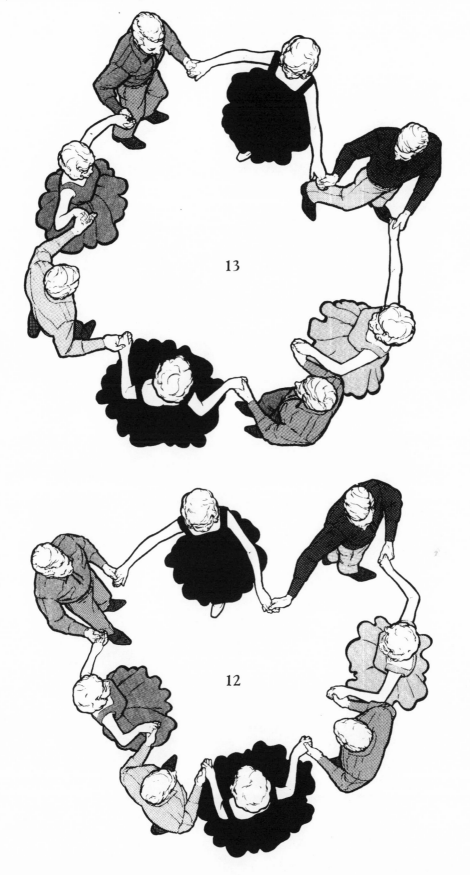

13

12

Figure 87. Rip and Snort (Frames 12 and 13 in a sequence of 13)

# Notes

# APPENDIX A

# What Is a Squaredance Fundamental?

*Essentials of the matter*

To get into the heart of the subject, we need to find answers to two questions.

1. How should we define the most fundamental unit of activity?

2. What procedures and maneuvers meet that definition?

*Aimed at experienced*

The material that follows is intended primarily for the knowledgeable and experienced caller/teacher or dancer, not the beginner. However, if the beginner should find it interesting and can grasp it, all the better for him, because knowing it will prevent his being caught up in the confusion currently so widespread. It is included as an appendix to this book because it explains the underlying body of thought upon which the book itself rests.

## PRELIMINARY DEFINITIONS

*Universal actions*

Before we go any further, we must define several things that are universal thruout squaredancing, being the all-embracing entities of action and control of action that make up this activity.

*Won't anger anyone*

Self-explanatory, these definitions are not likely to arouse antipathy in anyone, because none of them are a radical departure from previous unformalized thought and opinion.

*Not defined before*

Surprisingly enough, no one ever before has even settled upon a firm choice of terms to describe these things, much less formally defined any such sorely needed terms.

*Surprising situation*

It may seem strange that no one has done this previously. But there are perfectly good reasons why it is that no one has done so. One is that the process requires an almost incredible amount of the very hardest kind of work—brainrackingly deep thought. There are several other excellent reasons: Appendix D goes into them in some detail.

*No reflection*

Thus it is no reflection whatever on anyone in squaredancing that several things absolutely vital to continued progress in this activity have not been done sooner. The important point is that they finally have been done now.

*procedure* — a particular way of doing something; method of doing things.

*movement* — simplest type of change in the positions of the dancers.

*figure* — a set of movements; (sometimes) an action slightly more involved than a movement.

*maneuver* — a movement or figure.

*call* — an individual vocal expression (single word, group of words, or complete sentence) announced to the floor to direct one or more dancers to execute a certain maneuver or set of maneuvers bearing a single title.

*train of calls* — a coordinated succession of instructions delivered in sequence during the course of a single piece of music.

## What Qualifications Are Needed?

*Only its nature determines*

To return to the original question: What is a squaredance fundamental? Let us give a temporary answer by saying that *whatever* it may turn out to be when we delve into the matter, its being a funda mental is *not* determined by the extent or duration of its popularity.

*Nothing else*

Nor is it determined by the length or complexity of the call for it. Nor its smoothness, how easily it can be taught, nor anything else except its *nature*. It qualifies as a fundamental, or fails to qualify, strictly on the basis of its NATURE, *nothing else*.

*Primary concept of fundamentality*

Let's set that up in boldfaced type so we don't lose sight of it, because it is of primary importance and is the point where everyone has gone astray previously.

☞ **A maneuver's qualifying as a fundamental depends *only upon its NATURE*.** ☜

*Not just one level*

As this explanation progresses, the reader will see why it is that it is not feasible to establish a definition of one single, solitary level of fundamentality and call everything that meets it "a fundamental."

## The Character of Fundamentality

*Layers of bricks*

In brickwork or masonry one lays a row of bricks or stones, one beside another and with mortar between them. Such a layer is called a "course." By laying repeated courses, one on another, the person builds up a structure.

*Lowest tier a composite*

Now it turns out that in squaredancing there is a most-fundamental foundation course, all right, just as one would expect. But inextricably associated with it—directly on top of it and intertwined with it—is another course (a "first - and - a - half" course) not *quite* so starkly basal, but very nearly so, and still definitely fundamental.

Together these two interlaced courses make up an amalgamated (blended, or mixed) first or lowest course that comprises the fundamentals. Hereafter we will speak of these two courses as the lower and upper parts of the first or lowest course, of which they are the constituents.

## New Nomenclature

*"Fundamentals" includes two*

Exactly what does the word "fundamentals" comprise? Two brand-new expressions (as applied to squaredancing) that we will learn more about as we proceed.

*Rudiments in first course*

The word *rudiment* is one formerly extremely common in grammar schools. A composite dictionary definition of its general meaning is informative.

### GENERAL DEFINITION

*rudiment* — a first principle, element, or fundamental, as of a subject to be learned; fundamental skill taught or learned (as in elementary school); a first step.

And there we have a fine term answering one of our needs perfectly. The maneuvers and procedures (hereafter for the sake of simplicity often referred to collectively as simply "maneuvers") in the lower part of the mixed first course are aptly and descriptively designated *rudiments*.

*Rudiments are elements*

But what are we to call the maneuvers in the upper part of the mingled lowest course? As we can see in the definition above, every rudiment is an element. Let us examine a composite dictionary definition of the general meaning of the word *element*.

### ANOTHER GENERAL DEFINITION

*element* — a component, feature, or principle of something; basic part; one of the relatively simple parts of any complex substance or process; one of a number of distinct units or parts of which something is composed.

*Rest are other elements*

Hence we can accurately denominate the procedures and maneuvers lying directly atop those in the very lowest portion of the foundation course, and interwoven with them, as *other elements*.

*Reiteration of foundation*

At the very bottom of the whole structure we have *rudiments*, which are a special kind of element. Right on top of those special elements, and intertwined with them, we have some more elements that are for individual specific reasons not *quite* so rudimentary, but still fundamental. It is logical and sensible to call these *other elements*.

Thus the fundamentals of squaredancing are rudiments and other elements. Accordingly, whenever the expression "the fundamentals" occurs, those two things are what is meant. In equation form,

## Fundamentals = Rudiments + Other Elements

# RUDIMENTS

*Must define*

We have decided what we are going to call the constituents of our composite first course. Very well. Now we must arrive at a standard by which to determine whether a given maneuver meets the qualifications of a rudiment. That is to say, we must rigorously define precisely what we mean by the word *rudiment* as we intend to apply it in squaredancing.

IMPORTANT DEFINITION

*rudiment* — a least-complicated process for accomplishing a most-elementary desired result; any simplest and distinctly unique action(s) making up a fundamental unit of activity; a rudiment always is straightforward and unembellished.

*Crux of matter*

This is the central definition that is the core around which our entire structure is to be erected. Understanding it clearly is crucial to the whole business at hand. If the reader will study it diligently, just as we used to pore over knotty problems in school, he will find the effort richly rewarding.

*Profound concepts, few words*

A great deal is said in only a few words in this pivotal, starting-point definition on which hinges our complete scheme of systemization. For that reason considerable explanation will be necessary to make unmistakably clear exactly what is meant. It is suggested the reader hark back to the definition whenever he feels the need while reading thru the explanation and ruminating on it.

## QUALITIES OF THE RUDIMENT

*Accomplishes only one result*

A rudiment must not accomplish more than one desired result nor comprise more than one recognizable, identifiable unit or part. Theoretically, the specific result desired could be any one of hundreds of actions, changes or exchanges of position, and the like.

*In theory could be many*

Furthermore, each of these most-elementary desired results could in theory be performed in several distinctly different ways. Hypothetically, therefore, a very large number of rudiments could be devised.

*Most weeded out*

In actuality, however, it has been found by a process of elimination consisting of trial and (mostly) failure that only a relatively small number of rudiments are practicable, useful, and enjoyable.

*Status changes occasionally*

At present there are 51 active ones, plus two others currently dormant but apt to be revived at any time, for a total of 53. Later that figure may change.

*Won't be many more*

But it is doubtful there will be any radical increase, and it is entirely possible that some of the present rudiments might drop out of favor and be eliminated from the roster of active ones. However, they would still be rudiments, despite being dormant.

# ACCOMPLISHING THE DESIRED RESULT

*General and precise methods*

The mechanics of the process make up the exact or precise method employed, which may fall into any one of several categories of *general* methods of activity. The general categories are listed in Table I at the end of this appendix. Please examine that table carefully before proceeding any further.

The reader should understand that there is no direct relation between the groupings of rudiments in Table I and the order in which they and the other elements are grouped or introduced in *Squaredance Fundamentals*.

*Unique, but not necessarily sole, way*

Note carefully that a rudiment does *not* have to be the *only* way of accomplishing the particular desired result; there may be several. There may even be several that fall within the same category of general method.

But the *precise* method employed must be unlike any other in either the same or another general group. That is, it has to be plainly and unmistakably *different* from every other possible way of accomplishing that result.

*Simplest way*

Furthermore, the precise method used must be the very *simplest* way of accomplishing that result under the conditions imposed. Later we will talk about the significance of "under the conditions imposed." But right now we need to grasp exactly what is meant by the statement that it must be the simplest way.

*Rollaway illustrates*

Rollaway affords us a good illustration of this point. The most-elementary result desired in executing it is an exchange of position, but not direction of facing, by partners who start out standing beside each other and facing in the same direction. One of them (usually the lady) moves across in front of the other (usually the gent) to the other side of him. The manner in which the lady moves across is in a *rolling mode*.

## Ways *Not* the Simplest

### OUTLANDISH EXAMPLE

*Lady gymnast*

Now let us suppose the lady were an accomplished gymnast. Midway thru her rolling action, she could do something extraordinary. In a split second she could execute a "standing" forward somersault as she went.

*No interruption*

She could land in precisely the same attitude and position she would have been in at that moment had she not performed the stunt but simply continued in a regular Rollaway.

Without pausing even for a moment, and keeping perfect time with the music, she could resume her rolling action and complete the maneuver. Thus the only difference between this maneuver and a normal Rollaway would be her flip in the middle of it.

*Could be*

Admittedly this is rather farfetched and unlikely from the standpoint of practicality. Nonetheless, it is perfectly valid as an example, because it is feasible if the lady should have the gymnastic ability to carry it out.

# Appendix A

*Must include nothing not needed*

The point is that if she did do that, or *anything else that was not needed*, the maneuver would *not* be the simplest way of accomplishing the most-elementary desired result, for the method employed and the conditions imposed.

*Same for gent*

Neither would it be if the gent should perform some less astonishing but equally unnecessary motion or action, such as whirling full around as the lady was rolling, or suchlike. Now the reader can see why the last part of the definition states that "a rudiment always is straightforward and unembellished."

## Three Maneuvers, Same Result

Half Sashay, Rollaway, and Whirlaway are a trio of maneuvers that help in further understanding the definition of a rudiment. The same thoroughly elementary result previously described for Rollaway is desired in executing all three of them. That is an exchange of position, but not direction of facing, by partners who start out standing beside each other and facing in the same direction.

## DIFFERENT GENERAL METHODS

### Half Sashay and Rollaway

*Half Sashay in category four*

In Half Sashay the lady steps sideways to the left in front of the gent, who steps sideways to the right behind her. Each simply moves in a certain way in respect to the other. By referring to Table I, the reader can see that this puts Half Sashay in the category of general method number four (D).

*Obviously different*

Rollaway accomplishes exactly the same result as does Half Sashay, yet obviously is completely unlike Half Sashay in the way it does it. The dissimilarity is apparent because even the general methods employed are different.

*Rollaway in category five*

In Rollaway one dancer rolls across in front of the other to the other side of him. The two act in direct, active cooperation—including physical contact with each other.

Again referring to Table I, we see this makes Rollaway fall into category number five (E).

*Each simplest, both rudiments*

As already mentioned, it is easy enough to discern that these two maneuvers bear practically no resemblance to each other. And in addition, for the way it goes about doing so, each accomplishes the desired exchange of position in the most straightforward, uncomplicated manner possible, without extraneous motions or actions. Therefore both are true rudiments.

### Half Sashay and Whirlaway

Half Sashay and Whirlaway also fall into the separate categories labeled D and E (four and five), respectively. Consequently, their unlikeness is equally apparent, and the same things mentioned before hold true for them. However, it may seem there is little difference between Rollaway and Whirlaway.

# SAME GENERAL METHOD

## ROLLAWAY AND WHIRLAWAY

*Quite similar*

It is true these two look very much alike. One reason is that both employ the same general method. They both are doing something in direct, active cooperation—including physical contact—with another dancer.

*Even same mode, but different precise*

Moreover, the similarity is increased by the fact that in both of them the lady moves across in front of the gent *in a rolling mode*. Nevertheless, the precise actions differ appreciably. The explanation of the inescapability of different precise methods follows.

*Must consider conditions imposed*

As stated previously, to be a rudiment the precise method used in carrying out a maneuver must be the very simplest way of accomplishing some most-elementary desired result *for the conditions imposed*. The conditions imposed have to be considered because they have a pronounced effect upon the exact makeup of the precise method. In fact, they often are the dominant factor.

*Very influential*

This is clearly seen in the case of Rollaway and Whirlaway. Were it not for the conditions imposed, these two would be identical—one and the same maneuver. But the conditions imposed at the beginning and at the end of each *force* the precise methods employed within the rolling mode to vary enough that two separate maneuvers result.

*Conditions in Rollaway*

In Rollaway the beginning condition is that the pair have one arm around each other's waist. The ending condition is that they have the other arm around each other's waist. Under these constraints, the gent can simply start the lady into the roll with one arm and catch her with the other.

*Conditions in Whirlaway*

But in Whirlaway the pair are obliged to begin with one *handhold* and end with another. Imposing these conditions necessitates considerably more complicated action.

The dancers must maintain the original handhold halfway round the lady's course of travel, establish another grasp at that point while retaining the first hold momentarily, and then release the original hold and continue the second one as the lady moves into her final position. Thus there is plenty of difference distinguishing Whirlaway from Rollaway.

*Each simplest for own conditions*

Whirlaway is more involved than Rollaway, true. Nevertheless, if the dancers are constrained to start with the one handhold and end with the other, Whirlaway still is the simplest way of achieving the desired exchange of positions in the rolling mode employed within general method five.

And, as already demonstrated, Rollaway is the simplest way of achieving the same desired exchange of positions for the conditions imposed during *its* execution.

*Both rudiments*

Hence each is the simplest way of achieving the desired result for the precise method employed and the conditions imposed. Or, restating the latter part, ". . . for the precise method employed, *as largely determined by* the conditions imposed." Accordingly, both maneuvers meet the definition of a rudiment.

## RUDIMENT MAY DEPEND UPON RUDIMENT

One might note that a rudiment may be dependent upon (auxiliary to) another rudiment. For example, one cannot very well Shoot the Star or Throw in the Clutch unless he has previously been in an Allemande Thar.

*Wrongway Thar not rudiment*

We ignore Wrongway Thar, since as will be learned later, it is not a rudiment, but an other element, being merely a mirror image of Allemande Thar.

*Auxiliary to, but simplest way*

Obviously, then, both Shoot the Star and Throw in the Clutch are auxiliary to Allemande Thar. That fact notwithstanding, though, the following is true: For the way it goes about it, each is the very simplest way of discontinuing the backup star or of transforming it, as the case may be. Therefore both are just as much rudiments as the Allemande Thar itself is.

## OTHER ELEMENTS

*Definition*

At this point we know what a rudiment is and what maneuvers are rudiments. Now we need to know what an *other element* is. But that is easy; the worst is already behind us. Our definition of an *other element* is very simple and self-explanatory. Here it is.

*other element* — a fundamental unit of activity differing from a rudiment only in being in some manner a duplication of some rudiment.

## WHICH QUALIFY AND WHY

We also want to know which maneuvers qualify as other elements. They are the ones that almost, but not quite, meet the requirements for being a rudiment. One might denominate them " 'almost' rudiments." Here they are, categorized in respect to the way in which they duplicate some rudiment and thus fail to be rudiments themselves.

### MIRROR IMAGES

1. Balance Back
2. Lefthand Pullby
3. Seesaw
4. Seesaw Your Pretty Little Taw
5. Resashay
6. Left Star Thru
7. Turn Your Corner Under
8. Swat the Flea
9. Lefthand Star
10. Back by the Right
11. Wrongway Thar
12. Right Star Promenade

### VARIANTS

1. Alamo Style (Ring)
2. Split Corners
3. Grand Right and Left
4. Right Square Thru
5. Left Square Thru

### PACKAGES

1. Right and Left Thru
2. Two Ladies Chain

### REDUNDANCY

1. Allemande Left

# Explanation of Categories of Other Elements

### MIRROR IMAGES

These are exactly what their name implies—maneuvers that are identical with some other maneuver except for being reversed, right to left, the way the "parent" maneuver would appear when seen in a mirror placed at the appropriate position.

### VARIANTS

Each of these is a modification of some parent maneuver. For example, an Alamo Style (Ring) is in arrangement nothing more than an Ocean-Wave Line bent around and joined so as to form a special kind of circle or ring.

### PACKAGES

The packages of elements in group three are included as other elements because each package has been accorded the status of a single element by time-honored usage.

### REDUNDANCY

Allemande Left is a redundant form (a duplication) of Left Forearm Swing (or Left Hand Swing) under another name. Nowadays, unless it is executed with a Floatout (as, regrettably, it seldom is), it is functionally no different from any other Left Forearm (or Hand) Swing.

*Could argue*

One could argue in good logic that since one maneuver now is identical with the other, Allemande Left does not deserve to be included as a separate entity.

*Only apparently logical*

Despite its seeming logic, such an argument would be preposterous. The reason is that it ignores an extremely powerful point in favor of the distinctness of Allemande Left.

*Unique regardless*

That is the fact that a hundred years and more of squaredancing have firmly established this most-performed of all maneuvers as a unique element, regardless of *how* it is performed. Functionally it may be no different now from any other Left Forearm (or Hand) Swing, true. But in nomenclature and in its vital role as the veritable "backbone of squaredancing" it certainly is.

# More About the Characteristics of Fundamentals

*Holds for both*

The reader should bear in mind that whatever is said here in general about a rudiment holds true also for an other element, which really is nothing more than an " 'almost' rudiment."

*Must be workable*

A usable rudiment is a most-elementary maneuver (or procedure) that is practicable—that can be made to work. It does not have to have been used over a period of many years.

In fact, it does not have to have ever been used at all. However, it is exceedingly unlikely that any feasible ones would have been neglected amid the feverish search for "new basics," real or bogus.

*Must also be enjoyable*

But there is one other characteristic a maneuver has to have if it ever is to gain acceptance and actually be used. It must be not only workable, but also *enjoyable*.

*Unsuccessful candidates*

There are literally hundreds of changes and interchanges of position, and suchlike, that appear to be feasible but have been tried and found to be either 1) not workable, or 2) workable, but not enjoyable.

One might call these "unsuccessful-candidate" rudiments, because they never made the grade in acceptance.

### Dormant rudiments

There are others that have been used for awhile, then have fallen by the wayside. These could be called "defunct" rudiments. But "dormant" is a better word, because no one can say with certainty that they will not at some time enjoy a revival of favor.

### Rudiment forever

As for a given maneuver's qualifying as a rudiment while dormant, it makes no particle of difference whether the maneuver is currently popular or not. Once it has "established its credentials" as a workable rudiment, it remains such forever, regardless of its status.

### Current rudiments

Finally, there are those rudiments that are currently being used at any given time. These, together with the currently popular other elements accompanying them, are what probably will commonly be referred to as simply "the" fundamentals. But as just pointed out, their roster is subject to change from time to time, though not at all frequently. Therefore a more accurate title would be *current* fundamentals.

## ANOTHER NEW TERM: *CLASSIC*

### New but needed

There is a fine term that is badly needed by the squaredancer. Though it has been used in rounddancing, it has never been used before in squaredancing. But if adopted, it can go a long way toward helping to clear up confusion. It is the word *classic*.

### What a classic is

A classic of any kind is an individual example of that kind that endures in acceptance and popularity thru a considerable period of time. And in this sense the word *standard* could be used just as well as *classic*, but one or the other should be chosen and used consistently by everyone.

This book recommends that for a given maneuver to qualify as a classic, it must have enjoyed reasonably widespread popularity for a period of five continuous years.

Some other period may eventually be adopted by a preponderance of policy-setting groups such as callers' associations, however.

### Fundamental and classic

It is imperative that one apprehend the difference between a fundamental and a classic or standard. A given maneuver quite possibly might qualify as both. But on the other hand it might qualify only as one or the other, and not both. There does not necessarily have to be any correlation whatever between them.

NOTE WELL that a single-titled grabbag figure composed of a number of fundamentals can be a classic just as well as a simple maneuver can, if it endures in popularity for the requisite length of time. (See the Glossary, pages *xii* and *xiii*, for a simple definition of a grabbag; a detailed explanation is given in Appendix B.)

# TABLE I

## CATEGORIES OF GENERAL METHODS OF ACTIVITY

### AND THE RUDIMENTS THEY EMBRACE

A. *Disposing one's bodily members in a certain manner.* Since little or no action is involved in them, these are procedures, rather than maneuvers.

1. Attention
2. Honors
3. Box Grip for Star Formation

B. *Positioning oneself (and usually moving) in a certain way in relation to others.* These would be procedures, rather than maneuvers, if the only thing involved were the placement of oneself in the proper position. However, the placement usually is merely a requisite for correctly performing the action. Generally the action is the real result desired.

1. Ordinary Straight Line
2. Ocean-Wave Line in the Conventional-Handclasp Mode
3. Ocean-Wave Line in the Lifted-Arms Mode
4. Circle
5. Promenade in Single File
6. Couple Promenade
7. Escort Stance
8. Single Arch
9. Double Arch

C. *Going from one place to another.*

1. Walk
2. Balance Up

3. Promenade Alone
4. Turnback
5. Forward (Up) and Back

D. *Moving in a certain way in respect to others.*

1. Rollback
2. Weave the Ring
3. Split the Ring
4. (Go) Round One (or Two, or Other Number)
5. Pass Thru
6. Cross Trail
7. Dive Thru
8. Do-Sa-Do
9. (Walk) All Around Your Lefthand Lady
10. Half Sashay
11. Resashay, (Go) All the Way Round

E. *Doing something in direct, active cooperation—including physical contact—with another dancer.*

1. Righthand Pullby
2. Forearm Swing with Elbow Grip
3. Forearm Swing with Forearm Grip
4. Hand Swing
5. Waist Swing

6. Wheelaround

7. Backtrack

8. Rollaway

9. Whirlaway

10. Right Star Thru

11. California Twirl

12. Box the Gnat

13. Courtesy Turn, Right-and-Left-Thru Entry

14. Courtesy Turn, Two-Ladies-Chain Entry

15. Courtesy Turn, Do-Paso Entry

F. *Doing something in direct, active cooperation—including physical contact—*

*with another dancer as participants in the more general activity of a larger group.*

This is a logical extension of category five.

1. Allemande Thar

2. Shoot the Star

3. Left Star Promenade

4. Spread the Star Out Wide

5. Hub Backs Out, Rim Goes In

G. *Participating directly in a group activity.*

1. Righthand Star

2. Back by the Left

3. Throw in the Clutch

4. Break to a Line

5. Rip and Snort

# APPENDIX B

# What the Basics Are

In commerce an inventory is a descriptive list of the number and value of articles on hand for practical, beneficial *use* (meaning, usually, sale). Similarly, in squaredancing the basics are the dancer's inventory of simple, uncomplicated maneuvers needed for use in smooth, enjoyable dancing that is not a memory test.

*Equation*

Now that we know what the fundamentals are and what a classic is, let us see what the basics are.

## Basics = All the Fundamentals + a Few Especially Useful Simple Classic Packages

*Will scrutinize*

To make sure we understand the above equation fully, we will examine its components in detail.

*First part firm*

The makeup of the first item on the righthand side of this equation—the fundamentals—is hardly open to question. It has been exhaustively proved in the preceding part of this dissertation (in Appendix A) that at present there are no more than 73 of them.

*Second part arguable*

But the exact identity of the constituents of the second item on the righthand side of the equation is a different matter. It can be argued at length among individuals, and doubtless it will be. What gives rise to the room for argument will be discussed presently.

## FUNDAMENTALS, CLASSICS, BASICS

*Fundamentals and classics*

There are quite a few classics. Some of them are fundamentals; many are not. Conversely, most fundamentals are classics, but a few are not.

In addition, practically any classic maneuver that is a *single* activity unit almost *has* to be a fundamental, because of its very nature. In theory there might be those that were not. But in actuality any such maneuver almost surely would already have lost all unneeded features and achieved the purity of a fundamental.

*All fundamentals are basics*

We can see from the equation above that by definition *all* fundamentals are basics, regardless of whether they are classics (single ones, of course) or not. And as we have just observed, there is little room for the classic singles to be anything *but* fundamentals, hence basics. Consequently, we will ignore the single classics and focus our attention on the classic packages.

## CLASSIC PACKAGES

*Reason for room for argument*

As stated previously, there is room for argument concerning the exact identity of the constituents of the second item on the righthand side of the equation given above.

The reason is that three factors must be considered in regard to each candidate package. They are as follows.

1. Longevity and widespreadness, to qualify the package as a classic.

2. Degree of simplicity, to establish that the package is in fact a *simple* classic.

3. Usefulness of the packaged components; it must be greater than that of those same components unpackaged.

All three of these considerations are subject to at least some degree of opinion. They are discussed at length in the following paragraphs.

### LONGEVITY AND WIDESPREADNESS

*No hit parade*

There is no squaredancing "hit parade" type of popularity rating based on continual sampling of the extent of preference and popular acceptance of maneuvers used in the activity.

*Need history to prove*

And unfortunately, a history compiled from the records of such a popularity-sampling poll is about the only way in which one could positively, absolutely prove that a given package maneuver really had been reasonably widely popular during the five continuous years (or other period that is eventually adopted by policy-setting groups) required to qualify it as a classic. Therefore this factor is very much open to debate. And it will remain so until a reliable, continuing method of popularity rating is instituted and has been in operation for at least five years.

### DEGREE OF SIMPLICITY

*Easiest to evaluate*

This is the factor least difficult to evaluate. By means of the techniques of analysis brought forth in these dissertations, it is a fairly easy matter to dissect any package and find out how many fundamentals it comprises.

If it contains more than three fundamentals, it is not a simple package, so cannot be a basic. Thus there is little room for argument on this point.

### USEFULNESS

*Point most open*

This is the point most open to individual opinion. But there is a standard by which to judge. It is as follows.

*Criterion*

*Can the fundamentals composing the simple package be called individually fully as handily and as smoothly as can the pack-*

*age name along with "helper" calls?* (Helper calls are defined later in this appendix.)

*Has to be more useful*

If they can, then even though the simple package may be a classic, it still is not —in and of itself, *as a unit*—particularly and especially useful. That is, it is not more useful than the unpackaged individual components.

In other words, it does not fulfill a real need that cannot be satisfied just as well by the individual components making it up. Therefore a simple package of this kind fails to qualify as a basic, even though it may be a classic.

EXAMPLE

*Candidate apparently difficult to judge*

Grand Square is an excellent example of a figure whose qualifications as a basic might appear to be questionable. It certainly qualifies on the first point, longevity and widespreadness. It has been universally popular for a great many years. And in actual fact it fully meets the requirement of simplicity, since it is composed of just one fundamental: Walk (forward and backward).

But it *appears* so complicated! People are going every which way at the same time. At least to the beginner, it appears almost like "fruitbasket turn over." Let us look into this matter a little more closely, though.

*Many simple actions at once*

First of all, the individual segments of action and their sequence really are not terribly involved, even though there are a lot of them going on at the same time. But the nub of the matter is the very fact that the separate actions of more than one individual *are* carried out simultaneously.

*Usefulness deciding factor*

For now we come to the factor of usefulness. This is the point that enables us to form a rational, supportable opinion. Because of the multiplicity of separate actions occurring simultaneously, it is almost impossible to call this figure completely and individually descriptively.

*Fulfills real need*

Hence this single-titled package does indeed fulfill a real need that cannot be satisfied just as well by the individual components making it up. Beyond any argument, it is *outstandingly* useful. Thus it meets all the requirements for being a basic and very definitely is one.

## CLASSIC GRABBAGS

*No grabbag a basic*

A grabbag is a package containing an inordinate number of fundamentals. Obviously, then, by definition no grabbag is simple; therefore no grabbag can be a basic.

*Quite a few classic grabbags*

But NOTE WELL that there are, in fact, a considerable number of classic grabbags in existence. To repeat, though: Because of their not being *simple* packages, none of them ever can qualify as basics, regardless of how widespread their popularity and how long it continues.

*May like and want to know*

Certain dancers (perhaps great numbers of them) may consider a particular classic grabbag very nice to have as part of their repertoire. If they want to add it to their accomplishments, that is fine, for by doing so they improve their competence as squaredancers.

*Still not a basic*

Nonetheless, if the figure contains enough components (fundamentals) to qualify for the designation "grabbag," it never can be a basic. And to call it that— or even to think of it as such—is an error tending to lead one back into confusion.

*Universal but undesirable*

In similar manner, the practically universal expression "basic fundamental" should be avoided. Even in the nomenclature used until the present time, such a phrase was redundant and unneeded. But now that we have clearly distinct definitions for these two terms, use of such a lame expression is doubly imprudent, because it tends strongly to drag one's thought processes back down into disorder.

*Most use helper calls*

It is noteworthy that most callers conform to a standard practice in connection with the more complex grabbags. Unless the caller is completely insensitive to the needs of the dancer (and few are), he usual-ly follows the call for the grabbag with "helper" calls (mentioned earlier, in the standard for usefulness).

*What helper calls are*

A helper call is an extra, additional call delivered after (usually) a grabbag call to make up for the lack of instruction in the grabbag call and help the dancer know what he is supposed to do.

*Classic simple packages*

There are a relatively few classics that are simple packages made up of two, or at most three, fundamentals. To emphasize this extremely important point one more time: These particular packages are the *only* ones that are eligible for consideration as possibly being basics. Typical examples are Do Paso, Dixie Chain, and Substitute.

*Can be called descriptively, but*

These can be called completely descriptively. But usually it is more convenient and smoother to call them by their package names.

However, that is not to say, though, that the caller does not oftentimes call at least some of the fundamentals composing such a package, *in addition*, as helper calls.

*Example concerning Do Paso*

A good example of this technique is the almost universal practice, after announcing Do Paso, of calling in addition "Partner left and corner right," just to help the dancer along and make sure he does the right thing. Of course these extra instructions also serve as patter (filler material) in the calling and help to make it smooth-flowing.

## PROSPECTS FOR THE FUTURE

*Basics always will vary more*

A certain amount of inexactitude is introduced by the considerations of longevity, simplicity, and usefulness. As a consequence, the roster of basics never can be as clearcut and uniform as that of the fundamentals.

*Views of individuals*

That is to say, many individuals still will have ideas that differ from those of other persons in regard to the qualifications of certain maneuvers as basics. And both will have legitimate arguments to cite in support of their stand.

*But not as much as before*

But despite the difficulties, the various lists of basics compiled by one person and another should not in the future differ as wildly as they have in the past. The reason will become clear shortly.

*Chaos previously*

Until now any grabbag call—however hideously intricate it might be—invariably has been instantly hailed as "the latest basic" and immediately added to many persons' lists of basics.

*Reason for chaos*

The reason for this condition is that until now no one has really understood just what a fundamental was, the relationship of a fundamental to a classic, of a classic to a basic, and the like.

*Guidelines established*

But now guidelines for evaluation have here been established. The understanding provided in this treatise should help greatly toward doing away with the pernicious practice of establishing "instant basics."

*Will have to justify*

Henceforth a proponent of a "new basic" will have to present justification and support for his nomination. Accordingly, a much clearer picture should result, and a reasonable degree of standardization should be achievable.

# APPENDIX C

# Descriptive Calling: The Remedy for a Major Problem

## BACKGROUND OF THE PROBLEM

*Names used as calls*

Maneuver names often are used as calls. For instance, it is extremely common to hear such instructions as "Meet your lady with the old right hand; here we go—right and left grand." Of course the first part of this one is patter preparing the listening dancer for the call proper, which is ". . . right and left grand" (a variant name for Grand Right and Left).

*What caller is saying*

Thus it can be seen that although Right and Left Grand, our typical example, usually is a noun title for a maneuver, it very often is used as a call directing the dancers to perform that maneuver. When the caller uses it in that way, he really is saying "[Do a] right and left grand."

*Fundamentals' names descriptive*

The names of most of the fundamental maneuvers are descriptive of the actions constituting those maneuvers. Again Grand

Right and Left is a good example. Its name alone gives a fairly good idea of what is involved in executing it: alternate Righthand and Lefthand Pullbys around the ring.

*Scads of nondescriptive*

But what ideas are conveyed by, for instance, Bucket of Worms? What clues does the name Snorkel Thru supply? What help is provided by the ludicrous Zip Code? None whatever. For these names, and a host of others like them, do not describe the maneuvers they are intended to instruct the dancer to perform. Totally *non*descriptive as titles, they are just as nondescriptive when used as calls.

*Glamorous but useless*

It is true that they almost always are fanciful, whimsical, or colorful—perhaps all three. But that is about the only good thing one can say for them. They are an abomination, buzzing around the dancer's (and the caller's) head like swarms of obnoxious insects.

## DESCRIPTION OF THE PROBLEM

*One call, several maneuvers*

A considerable percentage of the calls the dancer receives on the floor today are nondescriptive. Even worse, a single such

call often directs the dancer to perform not just one, or perhaps two or three, fundamental maneuvers (activity units), but four, five, or even more of them.

*Infinite number*

Because there are so many calls of this kind, all thought of and referred to as "basics," the dancer gets the idea there are almost an unlimited number of distinctly different fundamentals that he must be familiar enough with to recognize the call for and be able to perform within moments from the time he hears the call.

*No fun, quits*

Eventually he forms a conclusion. He decides that any activity purporting to be recreation but requiring two computers in tandem to prevent his making a fool of himself *is not fun*. Disgusted, he usually quits squaredancing, departing with a bad taste in his mouth.

## SOURCE OF THE PROBLEM

*Just so many*

There are only a limited number of ways in which a dancer or group of dancers can "go from here to there" in the set, and a limited number of things they can do as they proceed.

*Most already exist*

Put more briefly, there are only a fair-ly small number of true fundamentals that are feasible and enjoyable. (See Appendix A for details in this regard.) The roster of fundamentals has remained stable for several years now. Therefore it appears that most of the fundamentals have already been devised.

## CAUSE OF THE PROBLEM

*Creative urge*

Nonetheless, many persons harbor within them a powerful creative urge. It is natural for them to want to give vent to this urge along lines they are most interested in and enthusiastic about. Hence many callers seek an outlet for it in coming up with what they consider something new in the way of calls.

*Think are creating*

As already mentioned, most of the fundamentals have long since been fully developed. But until now no one has known this to be a fact, since they did not even know what the fundamentals actually were.

Being unaware of these facts, callers interested in making up new things for the dancer have done something they thought to be creatively original, but that in fact was not.

*What some have done*

That is, without realizing or understanding what they truly were doing, they have selected numbers of fundamentals and arranged them in a particular order, then given the group a single fancy name.

*Strung together, packaged*

The fundamentals might be likened to beads. The universal procedure has been to thread fundamentals together in sequence, like a string of beads, then wrap them up, so to speak, into a neat package made attractive by "tying it with a pink ribbon" in the form of a catchy name for the whole bundle.

### "New basics"

Each and every specimen of this sort of thing is invariably heralded as "a new basic" as soon as it is hatched. But such monstrosities actually are about as basic as the reams of printout from a high-speed computer. Their constituents are simple, but their bulk (quantity) is formidable. To call them basic is to corrupt and pervert the word "basic."

### Can boast

These hodgepodges are simply an outlet for the ego we all have. They enable a caller to proudly say to the world "Look at me! I'm the fellow who invented the Snorkel Thru with a Scooby Doo—the newest basic!"

### Dancer suffers

The fact that 47 other "newest basics" were concocted on the same day is overlooked by all concerned except the dazed, bewildered dancer, who moans "Oh, no! Not another one! We can't remember them all now!"

### Flashy packages

These packages are enticing to many people. Their sole attractive feature is their snappy title. But it usually does indeed have a lot of "flash," as carnival operators say. Of course such bundles really are grabbags, because their names convey no inkling of their components. That is, the calls for them are nondescriptive.

### Mystery attracts

Being nondescriptive, they are in fact mystery calls. Oddly enough, however, their very inscrutability is what constitutes a powerful lure for a great many people. To these dancers and callers, a catchy title that they cannot fathom at first encounter has a tremendous amount of the glamour of the obscure.

### Psychology of it

The psychology is this: "If I don't understand it, then it must be only for those 'in on the know.' Knowing what it means must be a sign of distinction setting one apart from the less knowledgeable and marking one as a 'high-level dancer.'"

### Ultimate in "in"

One might be tempted to adapt an old vaudeville joke and remark that anyone could much more easily become a "high-level dancer" by simply taking the elevator to a dance hall on an upper floor.

Or more realistically, one could state with a considerable degree of seriousness that the ultimate in "in" calls is any that are spoken or sung in Sanskrit. Since it is a synthetic (artificial, constructed) literary language that no one ever spoke natively, *no* one would understand the calls until he had gone to the trouble of learning that exotic language.

### Simply a sham

What everyone overlooks, in the flush of satisafction at being able to feel superior to the common herd, is this: *Nothing whatsover has been gained.* Nothing useful, or helpful, or of service to the dancer has been added.

For encapsulating several fundamentals in a single flashy wrapping does not in any way contribute to the dancer's ability to recall and execute that set of fundamentals. On the contrary; it severely impairs his ability to do so, and to no good purpose, either. How much better to refrain from playing magician with mystery calls and instead call descriptively.

*Better for both*

Such calling is not just easier to dance to. It also is fully as advantageous for the caller, too. It is easier for him to do, and it provides him with a far simpler, sounder base on which to choreograph (arrange) trains of calls.

## ANSWER TO THE PROBLEM

*Definition*

What is descriptive calling? Here is a formal but very simple definition of it.

*descriptive calling* — that employing only calls for basics.

*Foremost advantage*

The beauty of descriptive calling is this: The dancer receives a smooth, continuous flow of instructions in the form of names representing activity units plenty small enough for him to recognize, recall the details of, and perform without difficulty. Without having to try to be a human computer with a ten-zillion-digit memory bank, he can dance competently to anyone anywhere who calls descriptively.

*Only a few*

There are only 73 fundamentals to learn, and the simple classics composed of combinations of two or three of them are not very numerous. Hence the total number of basics is not great.

*Adequate for anything*

Absolutely anything can be done with the basics that can be done by lumping those same simple individual maneuvers into a few outrageously large bundles and giving each collection a fancy title that affords the listener no hint about what all is included in the package.

*What grabbing calls are*

And that is all a grabbag is—a number of small activity units assembled into one very large activity unit dubbed with a glamorous but unfathomable name.

## THE DANGER WE FACE

*Back to prompters*

Carried to its ultimate absurdity, grabbag calling will bring us full circle, back to the days when squaredancing did not have callers, but prompters. At that time there were only a handful of dances in existence, and the dancers knew them all by heart. Each consisted in a complete train of

maneuvers performed during the course of a single piece of music.

*Fired gun, fiddled*

Usually the prompter was also the fiddler, who furnished all or part of the music. Virtually all he did as a prompter was to "fire the starting gun"; then he turned his attention to his fiddling. Each whole dance was one huge grabbag, but the dancer had no problem, because there were so few dances, and the contents of all of them were well known by everyone.

*Way we are headed*

If the contents of individual grabbag calls continue to expand, soon we will have much the same situation again. But it will be different in one respect, causing it to be very bad this time. For there will be innumerable grabbags—so many that no one can hope to learn and remember the contents of them all.

*Won't be many dancers*

At that time there won't be any more people squaredancing than there were during the days of the prompter, despite a population eight or ten times as large.

*Cause of enjoyment*

The reason is that most of the extraordinary enjoyment offered by modern squaredancing results from the constant but reasonable challenge presented by a string of small activity units whose order is not known in advance. When this challenge vanishes from the pastime, so will the people. That will occur if descriptive calling is substantially replaced by sheer memorization of the contents of hundreds of grabbags.

*Not likely to happen*

This condition is not likely to come to pass in its entirety. Nevertheless, we have already approached it to a dismaying degree—closely enough that it behooves us to do something about matters before squaredancing suffers any more from this hurtful influence.

## WHAT LIES AHEAD

*Don't have to know*

One does not have to know precisely what the true basics of squaredancing are to call descriptively. Till now, no one has known for sure. Yet here and there a few hardy souls have ignored the clamor and the glamour surrounding grabbag calls and have stayed with calls that were descriptive.

*Didn't know formally, but felt*

None of these people ever sat down and consciously, purposefully figured out what the basics really were. But they had a keen "feel" for what had real substance to it and what offered only tinsel and flash. If it was not substantial, they refused to use it. Almost instinctively they were able to sort the wheat from the chaff and reject the latter.

*Most popular*

It is heartwarming to realize that a few people were able to stick with the genuine and avoid the deceptive thru exercise of little more than common "horse sense." And incidentally, it is worthy of note that these callers have in almost all instances enjoyed a steady, unwavering popularity thruout their calling careers.

*Need formal knowledge*

But to do the very best in calling descriptively and have positive assurance one is avoiding useless material, it is necessary to have a clear understanding of what a fundamental is, which maneuvers are basics, and the like. One can go only so far on intuition and common sense. Beyond that he must have a body of accurate, systematized knowledge available to him to guide him in his course of action. That is, methodology has to replace the intuitive approach.

### Provides understanding

This book, particularly the dissertation in Appendix A, provides the complete information indispensable to anyone who would like to employ, as near as is feasible, only pure, unadulterated descriptive calls. In addition, it furnishes a mighty weapon with which one can refute the shallow arguments often brought forth in defense of grabbag calling.

### Grabbags will go

Descriptive calling will eventually supplant grabbag calling. It is inevitable that grabbags give way and descriptive calls triumph, because the latter are superior in every respect. When enough dancers and callers perceive this to be a fact, grabbag calling will disappear practically overnite.

### Balloon monster

Right now grabbag calling is an awesome monster apparently menacing the very continuance of squaredancing as an activity. But in actuality it is nothing more than a gigantic, fearsome-looking balloon.

This book is a weapon that can and will shoot holes in it. All the balloon has in it is a great deal of hot air. When that is let out, the dreaded monster will be seen for what it really is—a big sham that has no substance to it.

### Will run to get aboard

As soon as the dragon is slain, callers everywhere will awaken from the spell they have been under and will race to embrace the calling approach that satisfies to the fullest everyone concerned: descriptive calling.

### Dancers will flock in

When the time arrives that descriptive calling is considered normal procedure, instead of a strange practice indulged in by only a handful of eccentrics, a marvelous thing will occur. People will veritably batter down squaredancing's door, wanting in.

The reason will be this: they will be able to go to a club in New England, the Deep South, the Midwest, the Far West—anywhere at all in this country—and be able to thoroughly enjoy themselves while dancing competently with complete ease. Hearing no strange calls anywhere, they will be able to do this, and it will bring them in in droves.

### No worry about boredom

There is very little danger of the dancers' hearing the same trains of calls to the point of boredom. The only possible cause there could be for a monotonous sameness of calls would be laziness on the part of some callers in selecting their trains of calls, because there are an unlimited number of sequences in which 73 ingredients can be used.

### Can continue stringing

Callers everywhere can continue the very same process they enjoy so much today—stringing building-block beads in endless variety. Only instead of lumping several of them and giving the group a single fancy name, the callers will simply leave the beads as individual entities, without lumping them. The callers will enjoy themselves, and the dancers will be provided with never-ending profusion of variety.

### Nice challenge, no memory test

Every dance will be a challenge—not a memory test, but an enjoyable challenge demanding only alertness and attention to meet. The dancers will love it; they already do in the few places where it is offered to them.

# APPENDIX D

# Steps in the Creation of This Book

*Treatise explains*

The contents of this book rest upon a body of thought the particulars of which are explained in great detail in Appendices A and B. What is given here in Appendix D is a step-by-step account. It is of the procedure that was followed, once the basic philosophy had been arrived at, in finding a way out of chaos and structuring a rational, ordered system satisfactory for use by everyone concerned with square-dancing in any way.

*Anyone can give an opinion*

Anytime one deals with the fundamentals of anything, he is in deep water. Practically anyone who takes a notion to do so can sit down and rip off a glib, superficial dissertation, amounting to no more than an intuitive opinion, on the surface aspects of almost any subject, however complex.

*Bucket of worms*

But it is different if he is one of the few who actually give the matter a modicum of thought. Dipping beneath the surface, he discovers there a seething sea of snakes. Appalled, he almost invariably desists forthwith.

*Analysis unbelievably difficult*

It is only an infinitesimally small percentage of those in any field who have the inclination, the time, and the diligence to put in the fantastic number of hours of hard work (thought) necessary to resolve knotty subject matter and bring order out of disorder and confusion.

*Definitions absolutely essential*

A prime requisite for the process is to find or devise formal definitions of the terms one intends to use. If adequate ones are already in existence, they can be used. But if there are none, then one must make them up. If necessary, cut them from whole cloth. That is what the author did in this instance.

*First cut at analysis*

In order to construct definitions, though, it first was necessary to analyze the subject matter. To that end he dissected and closely examined dozens, scores, hundreds of figures to ascertain what activity units they were composed of. This effort alone demanded staggeringly large outlays of time and effort.

*Second cut at analysis*

Then he went back and investigated those activity units even more minutely. Each was scrutinized with a figurative electron microscope, so to speak, in an attempt to determine which of them appeared to be truly fundamental. All had to be sifted, sorted, weighed, and appraised from a number of aspects. This task required enormous amounts of almost unbelievably hard thought.

*Constructed definitions*

Next, on the strength of the insight and understanding gained thru that process, the author proceeded to make up his definitions. He cut them from whole, fresh cloth and tailored them to fit the needs of the problem. It was necessary to revamp them a slight bit as further study and deliberation made certain points clearer, but in the main the definitions proved sound as originally conceived.

### All have aversion

Making up the definitions was the hardest part of the whole project. The reason is that all of us are innately averse to getting formal and viewing in an impersonal, detached manner anything for which we have a warm affection.

### Psychology of repugnance

We are opposed to it in the same way we would be to talking about a human being (and especially a close friend) in terms of the market value of the chemicals making up his body. Or to seeing someone feed highly personal data into a computer to let the thing pick out a date or a mate for him. If we like something and enjoy it, we do not want to become cold and clinical in our thinking about it.

### Had to despite aversion

But that is precisely what *has* to be done if one is to make up formal definitions of anything. And formal definitions are absolutely essential to the process of developing sense and system from a jungle of unfounded opinion and intuitive feelings that long have passed for established order and arrangement.

### Author's stronger than reader's

Thus for the reasons mentioned, seeing squaredance terms formally, dispassionately defined may initially evoke a fairly sharp note of resentment in the reader. If so, rest assured the author had to face and overcome far stronger similar feelings while formulating those definitions. Yet he persevered, because he knew full well it simply had to be done, else the problem could never be solved.

### Third cut: testing against definitions

A further process had to be carried out before this book could result. After making up the definitions, the author was obliged to reexamine all the hundreds of activity units. Each had to be tested against the appropriate definitions to see which were indivisibly fundamental and what slot each of those fell into.

### The true building blocks?

There were 73 that emerged from the siftings and sortings. The final step was to take a hard look at them and apply the surest test of any system. That is, to ask the jackpot question: "Excluding novelties such as Boompsadaisy, can one really synthesize (put together parts so as to form a whole) any figure whatever, using only these 73 building blocks?"

### Experts say 'yes'

The author's carefully weighed answer was Yes, and it has since been supported by the considered opinions of two of the country's finest full-time professional callers. Of course there is always the possibility that someone may come up with something that cannot be synthesized from these 73. Another way of saying the same thing is that another true fundamental may be developed. It could happen, but the likelihood appears rather remote.

### Other sets could be developed

Along the same line: In any subject this complex, there are various ways, all valid, in which one could analyze and organize the material at hand. Conceivably, other definitions could be constructed and other systems built upon them. But till now, at least, no one has done so.

*Opportunity open*

If anyone can go thru as rigorous an analysis as the author did, on as sound a foundation, and come up with a more logical, workable, and *useful* set of fundamentals, then more power to him. But he had better be prepared to give good reasons for everything he has done and to defend his logic against all comers having all manner of objections. They will surely come his way.

# INDEX

# INDEX

Made in the USA